HALLELUJAH DIET

COOKBOOK

Transform Your Health with Simple, Flavorful, Plant-Based Diet Recipes for Weight Loss, a Healthier Gut, Prevention of Chronic Diseases, and Longevity

Eddy Beckett, MD

The content in this book is provided solely for general information purposes. While we make every effort to keep the information up to date and correct, we make no express or implied representations or warranties about the completeness, accuracy, reliability, suitability, or availability of the publication or the information, products, services, or related graphics contained in the publication for any purpose. Your reliance on such material is thus entirely at your own risk.

We shall not be liable for any loss or harm, including without limitation, indirect or consequential loss or damage, or any loss or damage deriving from loss of data or profits originating from or in connection with the use of this publication.

This publication may contain links to websites that are not under our control. We have no influence on the nature, content, or accessibility of other websites. The presence of any links does not constitute a suggestion or endorsement of the ideas expressed within them.

Every effort is taken to maintain the publication operational. Nevertheless, we accept no responsibility for, and will not be accountable for, the publication being momentarily unavailable owing to technical reasons beyond our control.

Table of Contents

CHAPTER 1: WHAT IS THE HALLELUJAH DIET?

The Hallelujah Diet stands as a beacon of plant-based nourishment, with its core focus resting on the consumption of raw fruits and vegetables, all rooted in the wisdom of a biblical passage. Its philosophy extends beyond mere sustenance, urging individuals to embrace whole foods and exclusive supplements, orchestrating a symphony of nutrients aimed at revitalizing the body's innate self-healing mechanisms. Remarkably, proponents claim this dietary regimen possesses the extraordinary capacity to reverse the progression of over 170 different maladies.

Yet, navigating the waters of the Hallelujah Diet requires an unwavering commitment, as it demands significant lifestyle recalibration and adherence to stringent guidelines.

However, amidst the rigors of this transformative journey, the program stands as a steadfast ally, offering an array of educational tools and enriching resources meticulously designed to empower individuals, facilitating both the initiation and perpetuation of dietary metamorphosis over the course of their lives.

Originating in the 1990s under the guidance of Reverend George Malkmus, this diet has garnered attention for purportedly improving personal health outcomes and fostering wellness in adherents.

At the core of the Hallelujah Diet are raw fruits, vegetables, and grains, constituting the foundation of meals while strictly eschewing prepared dishes, processed meats, and refined carbohydrates. Advocates of this dietary approach assert that embracing a predominantly plant-based and raw food lifestyle can result in heightened energy levels, bolstered immune function, and a reduced susceptibility to illness.

A distinguishing feature of the Hallelujah Diet is the incorporation of freshly squeezed vegetable juices, acclaimed for their abundance of vital nutrients believed to support optimal health. Proponents of the diet advocate for maintaining an alkaline pH within the body, contending that acidic environments are conducive to disease proliferation. Additionally, nuts and seeds are permitted in moderation, complementing the intake of fruits and vegetables.

Beyond its focus on physical well-being, the Hallelujah Diet underscores potential psychological and spiritual benefits. Aligned with its holistic philosophy, the diet discourages the consumption of caffeine, processed sugars, and artificial additives, emphasizing a natural and unadulterated approach to nourishment.

While the Hallelujah Diet resonates with individuals prioritizing their health and wellness, prospective adherents are urged to exercise caution and consult healthcare professionals before embarking on this dietary journey. It is imperative to ensure adequate nutrient intake and overall health maintenance under the guidance of medical experts, particularly considering the restrictive nature of the diet.

In summary, the Hallelujah Diet represents a compelling dietary paradigm emphasizing the transformative potential of plant-based, raw nutrition in fostering optimal health and well-being. As interest in holistic health approaches continues to grow, the Hallelujah Diet offers a holistic framework for individuals seeking to cultivate vitality and longevity through mindful dietary choices.

The diet's historical background or the historical context of the diet.

During the latter part of the twentieth century, there emerged a notable surge in the popularity of alternative medicine and dietary philosophies, setting the stage for the emergence of the Hallelujah Diet. Reverend George Malkmus, the creator of the Hallelujah Diet, embarked on a personal journey towards a plant-based diet rich in raw foods in the early 1990s, experiencing significant improvements in his health as a result.

Inspired by his transformative experience, Malkmus began sharing his dietary principles with others, eventually formalizing them into what is now known as the Hallelujah Diet.

This period witnessed a proliferation of alternative dietary approaches and lifestyle choices, driven by a growing awareness of the potential health benefits associated with food selection. Amidst this backdrop, the Hallelujah Diet emerged as an advocate for the belief that a diet centered around raw, plant-based foods, including abundant vegetables, fruits, and grains, could confer significant health advantages.

The resurgence of interest in natural, whole foods during the late twentieth century reflected a broader societal shift towards skepticism of processed and artificially enhanced foods. The Hallelujah Diet, characterized by its emphasis on "natural" and plant-based eating, resonated with individuals seeking to distance themselves from manufactured and heavily processed food products.

Furthermore, the narrative surrounding the Hallelujah Diet acquired added depth due to its connection to Reverend Malkmus' religious background. Marketed as more than just a dietary regimen, the Hallelujah Diet was promoted as a holistic way of life capable of enhancing not only physical health but also spiritual and emotional well-being.

The enduring appeal and continued adherence to the Hallelujah Diet serve as a testament to the enduring popularity of plant-based, holistic dietary approaches within contemporary health and wellness circles. Despite evolving trends and shifting cultural attitudes towards health and nutrition, the foundational principles of the Hallelujah Diet remain relevant, affirming the enduring relevance of plant-centric lifestyles in promoting overall health and vitality.

Advantages of the dietary regimen

The Hallelujah Diet is renowned for its focus on plant-based and raw foods, a dietary philosophy that advocates argue may offer numerous health benefits. Central to this approach is the belief that consuming a well-rounded diet rich in nutrients is essential for overall health and wellness. Advocates assert that the abundance of raw fruits, vegetables, and grains in the diet provides a concentrated and diverse array of antioxidants, minerals, and vitamins, all of which play crucial roles in supporting various biological processes within the body.

Among the purported advantages attributed to the Hallelujah Diet is its potential to bolster the immune system. Proponents of raw and plant-based diets argue that the high nutritional density of these foods contributes to improved health and heightened resistance to illness.

Furthermore, proponents of the Hallelujah Diet emphasize its alkaline-promoting nature as a means of safeguarding the body against acidic conditions. Advocates contend that maintaining a slightly alkaline environment within the body makes it less conducive for pathogens to thrive, thereby reducing the likelihood of developing various health ailments.

Many individuals also attest to the Hallelujah Diet's efficacy in weight management. For some, adhering to a plant-based diet that prioritizes whole foods while eschewing processed and calorie-dense options may facilitate weight loss and maintenance.

Moreover, proponents highlight the diet's positive effects on energy levels and cognitive function. By reducing reliance on caffeine and processed sugars, the Hallelujah Diet aims to enhance emotional and mental well-being as part of its comprehensive approach to overall health.

However, it's important to recognize that while the Hallelujah Diet may yield these benefits for some individuals, its effectiveness may vary depending on individual health status, lifestyle factors, and dietary preferences. Before embarking on any significant dietary changes, it is advisable to consult with healthcare professionals to ensure that nutritional needs are adequately met and overall health is safeguarded. By taking a personalized and informed approach to nutrition, individuals can optimize their well-being and vitality in alignment with their unique circumstances and goals.

CHAPTER 2: KEY COMPONENTS OF THE HALLELUJAH DIET

The Hallelujah Diet revolves around a plant-based dietary regimen, predominantly emphasizing the consumption of raw foods. At its core, this approach posits that ingesting uncooked produce is paramount for obtaining the full spectrum of vitamins, minerals, and antioxidants essential for optimal health. Advocates of the diet advocate that prioritizing whole, unprocessed foods in their raw state offers myriad health benefits.

Central to the Hallelujah Diet is the incorporation of freshly squeezed vegetable juices, heralded for their concentrated nutrient content and purported efficacy in cellular health and detoxification processes. Enthusiasts of the diet often underscore the importance of regular consumption of these fresh juices as a means of maximizing the diet's therapeutic benefits.

In addition to fruits and vegetables, the Hallelujah Diet permits, albeit in moderation, the inclusion of certain nuts and seeds, recognized as valuable plant-based protein sources essential for maintaining a balanced nutritional profile. With its foundational belief in the superiority of a predominantly raw and natural diet for human health, the diet strictly limits the intake of processed foods, animal products, and cooked items.

An integral tenet of the Hallelujah Diet is the maintenance of the body's pH at an alkaline level, purportedly fostering an environment less conducive to disease development. Proponents of the diet advocate for lifestyle choices that promote alkalinity, contending that acidic foods and beverages may disrupt the body's pH balance, potentially compromising health.

In summary, the Hallelujah Diet advocates for a plant-based eating pattern predominantly comprising raw foods, supplemented by the regular consumption of fresh vegetable juices and moderate intake of nuts and seeds. By eschewing processed foods, meat, and cooked meals, the diet aims to cultivate overall well-being by fostering a nutrient-dense, alkaline-forming dietary foundation conducive to natural, plant-based living.

The fundamental principles of dietary health

The foundational principle at the heart of the Hallelujah Diet revolves around the philosophy that embracing a predominantly plant-based, raw food lifestyle can serve as a robust cornerstone for fostering overall well-being. Proponents of this dietary philosophy firmly assert that raw fruits and vegetables are replete with an abundance of health-enhancing constituents, including essential vitamins, minerals, and antioxidants, all densely packed within their natural, unaltered forms. These vital nutrients are deemed essential for sustaining optimal health and vitality, supporting a myriad of critical bodily functions essential for life.

Central to the Hallelujah Diet is the incorporation of freshly squeezed vegetable juices into daily consumption habits. Advocates of this dietary regimen passionately extol the virtues of these rejuvenating elixirs, touting them as potent vehicles for delivering a plethora of vital nutrients crucial for promoting detoxification and cellular health. It is widely believed within the Hallelujah Diet community that a significant portion of the diet's health-promoting benefits can be attributed to the regular consumption of these invigorating beverages.

Furthermore, proponents of the Hallelujah Diet underscore the paramount importance of maintaining the body's pH levels within an alkaline range. The dietary guidelines meticulously outlined by proponents of this lifestyle aim to foster food choices that promote an alkaline state within the body, purportedly creating an internal environment less conducive to the development of various ailments. Embracing a diet abundant in alkaline-forming foods, such as fresh fruits and vegetables, while concurrently reducing the consumption of acidic fare, is advocated as a means to establish and sustain a harmonious internal equilibrium conducive to overall wellness.

Aligned with the broader health-conscious movement's emphasis on embracing natural, unprocessed foods, the Hallelujah Diet unequivocally rejects the consumption of prepackaged meals, refined foods, and animal products. Many adherents of this lifestyle report experiencing notable improvements such as alleviation of inflammation, enhanced digestion, and heightened levels of energy upon eliminating processed and refined foods from their dietary repertoire.

While individual responses to the Hallelujah Diet may vary, proponents of this lifestyle assert that embracing a plant-based, raw food dietary paradigm can yield a multitude of distinct benefits for physical health. These purported benefits include but are not limited to: supplying essential nutrients crucial for optimal bodily function, facilitating efficient detoxification processes within the body, and fostering an internal environment conducive to overall wellness and vitality. However, it is strongly advised to seek guidance from qualified healthcare professionals prior to embarking on any new dietary regimen to ensure nutritional adequacy and safeguard general health. Consulting with healthcare providers can provide invaluable assistance in navigating potential challenges and tailoring the diet to suit individual needs and wellness goals effectively.

The Diet's Spiritual Roots

The origins of the Hallelujah Diet are deeply intertwined with the spiritual beliefs of its founder, Reverend George Malkmus, whose own religious convictions served as the guiding light for this dietary approach. Malkmus, a devoted preacher, was inspired by the notion that aligning one's food choices with biblical principles could enhance both physical and spiritual health. According to proponents of the diet, adopting a plant-based and raw food lifestyle reflects an adherence to divine guidance outlined in sacred scriptures, thereby fostering holistic well-being.

For adherents of the Hallelujah Diet, the act of selecting plant-based and natural foods is perceived as a means of honoring the body as a sacred vessel, a temple entrusted to us by a higher power. By nourishing the body with wholesome, unprocessed foods, individuals demonstrate reverence for their physical form and strive to maintain its purity as an expression of gratitude for the gift of life.

Integral to the spiritual practice of the Hallelujah Diet is the incorporation of fasting, a time-honored tradition rooted in ancient practices of abstaining from certain foods for spiritual purification. Advocates of regular fasting assert that it serves to cleanse both the soul and the body, aligning with biblical principles of self-discipline and spiritual renewal.

Furthermore, the Hallelujah Diet emphasizes the importance of gratitude for the bounty provided by nature. Recognizing the miraculous origins of raw fruits, vegetables, and grains as gifts bestowed upon us by a divine source, individuals cultivate a deeper connection to the earth and its abundant offerings. In essence, the act of consuming these natural foods becomes an act of worship, strengthening the bond between humanity and the natural world.

In summary, the spiritual foundation of the Hallelujah Diet underscores the belief that embracing a plant-based, raw food lifestyle is not only conducive to physical health but also essential for spiritual well-being. Through practices such as fasting, reverence for natural foods, and stewardship of the body, individuals forge a deeper connection to their spiritual beliefs while nurturing their overall health and vitality.

CHAPTER 3: THE HALLELUJAH PLATE

The *Hallelujah Plate* is an essential part of the Hallelujah Diet, which provides a visual representation of the suggested food kinds and portion sizes for dieters to follow. People can use this symbolic plate as a practical tool to assist them stick to the diet ideals.

In most cases, you'll see three primary divisions on the Hallelujah Plate, one for each type of food. Raw, verdant, and colorful veggies should take up most of the meal. The value of eating a wide variety of raw veggies, which are high in antioxidants, vitamins, and minerals, is highlighted in this section.

To highlight the importance of eating raw, fresh fruits, the second part of the plate is set aside for them. In keeping with the Hallelujah Diet's emphasis on plant-based nutrition, fruits bring natural sugars, fiber, and extra vitamins to the diet.

Nuts and seeds are emphasized as a source of healthy fats and plant-based proteins in the third part, which also includes a tiny segment dedicated to them. The key is to keep your consumption in check, so feel free to enjoy these things in moderation.

In keeping with the tenets of the diet, the Hallelujah Plate suggests that people cut out processed foods, meat, and prepared meals. The Hallelujah Plate is a graphic representation of the required food groups and their proportions. It provides a simple and accessible guidance for those following the Hallelujah Diet to make balanced meals with a focus on plants.

Foods that are raw and derived from plants.

At the core of its nutritional philosophy lies the Hallelujah Diet, which revolves around the consumption of raw and plant-based meals. Advocates of raw food often assert that consuming foods in their uncooked state, particularly fruits and vegetables, preserves a higher concentration of essential nutrients. They argue that heating processes can diminish the nutritional content of foods by destroying vitamins and enzymes.

Plant-based diets, rich in vitamins, minerals, fiber, and antioxidants, offer a myriad of health benefits. These benefits include reduced inflammation and a decreased risk of chronic illnesses, attributed to the abundance of phytochemicals present in fruits and vegetables.

Experts on the Hallelujah Diet advocate for predominantly plant-based meals as the optimal means of fulfilling the body's protein, healthy fat, and carbohydrate requirements. While the diet prohibits the consumption of animal products, it encourages moderate intake of plant-based protein sources such as nuts, seeds, and legumes.

Moreover, the diet's emphasis on maintaining an alkaline environment within the body aligns with the consumption of raw and plant-based foods. Proponents of raw, alkaline-forming foods contend that they can help regulate the body's pH levels, thereby bolstering overall health and immunity.

Beyond the nutritional benefits, the Hallelujah Diet espouses a holistic approach to health, suggesting that consuming raw, plant-based meals can positively impact one's spiritual and emotional well-being. Advocates believe that these foods foster a deeper connection to nature and evoke a sense of purity, contributing to a more holistic state of nourishment for both the body and soul.

Ratios of Uncooked and Prepared Foods

All things considered, the Hallelujah Diet is built on the tenets of increasing nutritional intake, promoting a holistic approach to health, and sustaining an alkaline environment, the most important of which are raw and plant-based meals.

Supporters of the Hallelujah Diet argue that a large percentage of one's daily calories should come from raw, unprocessed produce. The diet usually suggests eating produce in its raw form, with the bulk of your servings coming from fruits and vegetables. An argument in favor of eating foods in their raw form is the idea that heating causes nutrients to be lost, especially heat-sensitive enzymes and vitamins. Many believe that the nutrients found in raw fruits and vegetables are more concentrated since they are in their most natural state and include a wider variety of vitamins, minerals, and antioxidants.

Although much of the Hallelujah Diet is based on raw foods, there are variants that permit a small quantity of prepared meals. If you're having trouble sticking to an all-raw diet, you may always include cooked grains and certain legumes in moderation. In order to maximize the consumption of pure and unprocessed plant-based meals, the Hallelujah Diet tends to favor raw foods over cooked ones.

Those who follow the Hallelujah Diet religiously claim that cutting out processed foods helps with digestion, gives you more energy, and improves your health in general. The theory goes like this: people may support their bodies' natural functioning and achieve maximum health by eating a diet richer in raw foods, which means they can absorb all the nutrients those foods provide. Keep in mind that the precise ratios within the diet might be impacted by personal tastes and tolerances, and that followers' adherence to these suggestio Upon comprehensive examination, it becomes evident that the Hallelujah Diet is grounded upon a multifaceted framework encompassing the augmentation of nutritional intake, the cultivation of a holistic approach to well-being, and the establishment of an alkaline environment, with particular emphasis placed on the consumption of raw and plant-based meals.

Advocates of the Hallelujah Diet posit that a significant proportion of daily caloric intake should be derived from raw, unprocessed produce. Central to the diet's philosophy is the recommendation to consume fruits and vegetables in their raw state, with an emphasis on maximizing servings from these sources.

Proponents argue that consuming foods in their raw form preserves vital nutrients, particularly heat-sensitive enzymes and vitamins, which may otherwise be compromised through cooking processes. It is widely believed that raw fruits and vegetables boast a higher concentration of nutrients in their natural state, offering a broader spectrum of vitamins, minerals, and antioxidants.

While the foundation of the Hallelujah Diet predominantly consists of raw foods, variations of the diet permit limited inclusion of prepared meals. Individuals encountering challenges adhering to an all-raw regimen are afforded flexibility to incorporate cooked grains and select legumes in moderation. However, the overarching principle of prioritizing the consumption of unprocessed plant-based meals remains paramount within the Hallelujah Diet.

Devotees of the Hallelujah Diet fervently assert that the elimination of processed foods facilitates enhanced digestion, heightened energy levels, and overall improvements in health. The underlying premise is rooted in the belief that by adhering to a diet abundant in raw foods, individuals can optimize their body's natural functions and maximize nutrient absorption, thereby fostering optimal health outcomes. It is important to note that adherence to the specific dietary recommendations may vary based on individual preferences and tolerances, and the precise ratios of food components within the diet may be subject

to adjustment to accommodate individual needs.
ns can vary.

Foods to steer clear of while following the Hallelujah Diet.

Emphasizing the exclusion of specific items believed to hinder optimal health and wellness stands as a central tenet of the Hallelujah Diet, a dietary approach that prioritizes whole, natural foods. At the forefront of this dietary philosophy is the avoidance of processed meals, which are viewed as detrimental due to their high content of processed sugars, artificial flavors, and preservatives. Within the framework of the

Hallelujah Diet, processed items are discouraged in favor of consuming more real, unprocessed foods sourced from nature's bounty.

Additionally, the Hallelujah Diet advocates for the elimination of animal products from one's dietary intake. This includes items such as eggs, dairy products, and meat, as proponents of the diet assert that a plant-based lifestyle aligns more closely with its principles. Accordingly, the emphasis is placed on increasing the consumption of fresh fruits, vegetables, and grains while reducing reliance on meat and dairy products.

Raw foods are highly encouraged within the Hallelujah Diet, with a preference for uncooked items over heat-treated alternatives. Many adherents of the diet eschew cooked meats, steamed vegetables, and other heat-processed foods, citing concerns that cooking may diminish their nutritional content. Thus, the diet advocates for the consumption of raw, uncooked foods to maximize nutrient intake and preserve their natural goodness.

Furthermore, the Hallelujah Diet discourages the consumption of caffeine-containing beverages, including coffee and certain types of tea. Instead, the diet recommends opting for herbal teas devoid of caffeine, aligning with its overarching principles of promoting a plant-based diet.

Added sugars, particularly refined sugars, are also discouraged within the Hallelujah Diet, reflecting a broader trend among health-conscious individuals to minimize processed sweets for the betterment of their overall health.

By adhering to these dietary guidelines, proponents of the Hallelujah Diet aim to cultivate what they term "optimum health" and a holistic sense of well-being through a diet rich in raw, plant-based alternatives. However, it is advisable for individuals to seek guidance from healthcare professionals before implementing significant changes to their diet, as individual dietary preferences and requirements may vary. Consulting with experts can help ensure that dietary modifications are tailored to meet individual needs and promote overall health and

wellness effectively.

CHAPTER 4: MANAGING NUTRIENT CONSUMPTION

Due to the inherent challenges in obtaining adequate nutrients strictly from plant sources, the Hallelujah Diet emphasizes the crucial importance of maintaining a well-balanced dietary regimen. In order to ensure an abundant array of nutrients, including vitamins, minerals, and antioxidants, the dietary guidelines advocate for consuming a diverse spectrum of fresh fruits and vegetables, representing the colors of the rainbow. This varied palate is deemed essential for providing the body with the essential nutrients necessary for optimal health and well-being.

In addition to vegetables and fruits, the Hallelujah Diet incorporates nuts and seeds in modest quantities, aiming to deliver protein, healthy fats, and additional vitamins to the dietary regimen. This inclusion of plant-based protein sources contributes to achieving a well-rounded nutritional profile, where striking a balance between caloric intake and protein and fat consumption is crucial.

An distinctive component of the Hallelujah Diet is the utilization of freshly extracted vegetable juices, which offer a concentrated source of nutrients that the body may find easier to absorb. Integrating this practice into one's dietary routine alongside consuming whole food meals is viewed as an enhancement for optimal nutrient absorption and maintaining nutritional balance.

To sustain a healthy nutritional equilibrium, adherents of the Hallelujah Diet are advised to attentively monitor their intake of vital nutrients such as vitamin B12, iron, calcium, and omega-3 fatty acids. In order to address any nutritional deficiencies that may arise from eliminating certain food categories, some individuals may be recommended to incorporate supplementation into their dietary regimen.

An integral tenet of the Hallelujah Diet revolves around maintaining the body's pH levels at an alkaline state. Adherents believe that a diet rich in alkaline-forming foods can facilitate this objective. By prioritizing consumption of fruits and vegetables while avoiding acidic foods, the diet aims to cultivate internal harmony, although the scientific evidence regarding the impact of dietary alkalinity remains debated.

Ultimately, ensuring adequate nutrient intake while following the Hallelujah Diet revolves around making informed food choices. Opt for a wide variety of plant-based foods to support overall health and wellness. As individual nutritional requirements may vary, consultation with healthcare professionals is recommended to devise a personalized dietary plan that suits your unique needs and goals.

The Hallelujah Diet emphasizes the importance of macro-nutrients.

The Hallelujah Diet offers an eating plan that prioritizes the careful management and equilibrium of carbohydrates, proteins, and fats, distinguishing itself from many other dietary approaches by its emphasis on the quality and composition of these macronutrients, rather than rigidly restricting specific food categories or meticulously calculating calorie intake.

At its core, The Hallelujah Diet espouses the belief that a healthy and sustainable dietary regimen can be achieved through mindful regulation of macronutrient consumption. Understanding the role of each macronutrient in contributing to overall nutrition is deemed essential for attaining optimal health and performance outcomes.

The dietary framework of The Hallelujah Diet suggests the adjustment of carbohydrate, protein, and fat proportions according to individual health and fitness objectives. For instance, individuals aiming for weight loss may opt to lower their carbohydrate and fat intake, while those striving to build muscle might increase their protein consumption accordingly.

To facilitate the monitoring of daily macronutrient intake, The Hallelujah Diet commonly employs the use of macro calculators or mobile applications. This practice of tracking food intake is recognized for its benefits in promoting weight management, enhancing athletic performance, and fostering overall health by raising awareness of food choices and portion sizes.

One of the key advantages of The Hallelujah Diet lies in its adaptability to diverse lifestyles and eating habits. Unlike some restrictive dietary plans, it does not prescribe specific meals or meal plans, allowing individuals the flexibility to consume foods they enjoy and avoid those they prefer not to include. This adaptability may enhance adherence to the diet over the long term.

Despite its flexibility, The Hallelujah Diet underscores the importance of prioritizing the quality of food choices within each macronutrient group. Opting for whole, nutrient-dense foods over processed or unhealthy options is advocated for achieving optimal health outcomes. Additionally, regulating portion sizes remains essential, particularly for individuals seeking weight loss.

The modifiability of macronutrient ratios within The Hallelujah Diet makes it a valuable tool for individuals seeking a systematic approach to healthy eating and a deeper understanding of how macronutrients function in the body. Consulting with a certified dietitian or nutrition specialist prior to embarking on the diet is recommended to ensure alignment with individual health and fitness objectives.

In its entirety, The Hallelujah Diet embodies a methodical and evidence-based approach to nutrition, offering individuals the flexibility to adjust their dietary habits to meet their specific needs and goals effectively. Through informed decision-making and personalized guidance, individuals can harness the potential of The Hallelujah Diet to optimize their health and well-being.

Ways to Obtain Essential Vitamins and Minerals

A fundamental pillar of the Hallelujah Diet lies in the comprehensive acquisition of essential nutrients exclusively from plant sources. Embracing raw fruits as a cornerstone, this dietary approach taps into their inherent wealth of diverse vitamins and minerals, including potassium, vitamin C, and antioxidants. Particularly prized are the vitamins abundantly present in citrus fruits, berries, and tropical varieties, renowned for their role in fortifying cellular integrity and bolstering immune function.

Elevating the nutritional quotient of the Hallelujah Diet is the incorporation of leafy green vegetables, esteemed for their rich reservoirs of vitamins A, K, and folate. From robust contenders like kale, spinach, to collard greens, these verdant powerhouses furnish indispensable nutrients like iron and calcium, indispensable for fortifying skeletal health and ensuring optimal blood oxygenation.

Furthermore, nuts and seeds emerge as pivotal contributors to the Hallelujah Diet's nutritional tapestry, serving as wellsprings of essential elements. Almonds, with their copious reserves of magnesium and vitamin E, and flaxseeds, endowed with ample fiber and omega-3 fatty acids, underscore the diet's commitment to fostering a balanced nutritional profile through the judicious incorporation of these plant-based protein sources.

Cruciferous vegetables, such as cauliflower and broccoli, take center stage in the Hallelujah Diet's nutritional symphony, offering generous doses of vitamins C and K. Beyond their vitamin bounty, these cruciferous marvels harbor sulfur-containing compounds, believed to exert beneficial effects on bodily well-being, further amplifying the diet's holistic health strategy.

An intriguing facet of the Hallelujah Diet manifests in its distinctive practice of imbibing freshly squeezed vegetable juices. These elixirs serve as potent vehicles for delivering a concentrated burst of essential vitamins and minerals, meticulously extracted from a medley of vegetables brimming with nutrient richness.

While the Hallelujah Diet fervently advocates for the holistic nourishment derived from plant-based sources, it acknowledges that some individuals may opt to supplement their dietary intake with additional minerals or vitamins. As part of a comprehensive approach to addressing potential nutritional gaps and ensuring a well-rounded nutritional strategy on the Hallelujah Diet, seeking guidance from healthcare specialists is advised. Through collaborative engagement with healthcare professionals, individuals can tailor their dietary regimen to optimize nutritional adequacy and promote overall well-being within the framework of the Hallelujah Diet.

Incorporating dietary supplements into one's nutritional regimen.

The Hallelujah Diet adopts a versatile and prudent stance regarding the utilization of supplements. While emphasizing the abundance of essential nutrients available in a diverse array of plant-based, raw meals, the diet recognizes the inherent variability in individuals' nutritional requirements and acknowledges the potential for nutritional gaps to arise.

Acknowledging the importance of vitamin B12, primarily found in animal-derived foods, the Hallelujah Diet underscores the necessity of considering supplementation for adherents who may not obtain adequate amounts through dietary sources devoid of animal products. Given the pivotal role of vitamin B12 in nerve function and red blood cell production, ensuring sufficient intake is imperative to prevent potential health complications.

Furthermore, individuals with heightened iron requirements may find benefit in supplementing their diet with iron, another vital mineral that may be deficient in plant-based diets due to the lower absorption rate of non-heme iron from sources such as leafy greens and legumes compared to heme iron from animal products.

The absence of dairy products in the Hallelujah Diet prompts consideration of calcium supplementation, particularly for individuals who may not meet their calcium needs solely through plant-based milk alternatives and select leafy greens. While these sources offer some calcium, supplementation may be warranted for those with inadequate dietary intake.

Omega-3 fatty acids, renowned for their cardiovascular and cognitive health benefits, are commonly sourced from fish oil. However, adherents of the Hallelujah Diet who abstain from fish consumption may opt for algae-based omega-3 supplements as an alternative source to support their nutritional requirements.

It's essential to underscore that supplementation within the framework of the Hallelujah Diet is intended to be personalized. Thus, followers are encouraged to engage in discussions with healthcare professionals to assess their individual nutrient needs and determine the appropriateness of supplementation. While whole food consumption remains paramount within the diet's philosophy, responsible supplementation can serve as a valuable tool in addressing any potential nutritional deficiencies and promoting overall health and well-being.

The beneficial impact of the Hallelujah Diet.

Despite being reiterated countless times, the importance of consuming ample fruits and vegetables remains a cornerstone of optimal health. Regrettably, a significant portion of the population, particularly those residing in urban areas, consistently fall short of meeting recommended dietary guidelines in this regard. According to data from the Centers for Disease Control and Prevention (CDC), merely one in ten Americans attain the recommended daily intake of fruits and vegetables. Alarmingly, a mere 10% of individuals meet the daily target of two to three cups of vegetables, while a mere 12% fulfill the daily goal of one and a half to two cups of fruit.

In addition to the evident health benefits derived from increased fruit and vegetable consumption, meeting these minimal requirements has also been associated with a potential increase in life expectancy. Research suggests that adhering to a diet rich in fruits and vegetables correlates with a reduced risk of mortality from various causes, including heart disease and cancer. Notably, studies indicate that the mortality risk does not decline beyond a consumption threshold of five servings per day, thus underscoring the importance of aiming for this quantity.

Visualizing serving sizes can aid in achieving the recommended intake: one cup of fruit or vegetables is roughly equivalent to the size of a tennis ball. Strategically incorporating these servings throughout the day can facilitate meeting dietary goals, such as consuming one cup of fruit at breakfast and another during snack time, along with one cup of vegetables at lunch and two cups in the evening. Furthermore, combining fruits and vegetables can enhance their palatability and convenience, such as blending them into a smoothie with frozen berries or incorporating fresh fruit into salads and stir-fry dishes.

By adopting such strategies and conscientiously increasing fruit and vegetable consumption, individuals can enhance their overall nutritional intake and potentially improve their long-term health outcomes. Prioritizing the inclusion of these nutrient-dense foods in daily meals not only promotes physical well-being but also contributes to a proactive approach to health maintenance and disease prevention.

CHAPTER 5: TASTY RECIPES FROM THE HALLELUJAH DIET, BASED ON PLANT-BASED INGREDIENTS

HALLELUJAH DIET RECIPES FOR BREAKFAST

Spicy Cajun Hash on Grits

INGREDIENTS

11/2 cups low-sodium vegetable broth

6 to 8 cloves garlic, minced

11/2 cups dry stone-ground grits

1 cup chopped onion

1 cup chopped red bell pepper

1 cup chopped celery

1 cup chopped carrots

2 tablespoons salt-free Cajun seasoning

2 cups cherry tomatoes, halved

1 15-oz. can no-salt-added small red beans or kidney beans, rinsed and drained (11/2 cups)

1 cup frozen cut green beans

Sea salt and freshly ground black pepper, to taste

2 tablespoons chopped fresh parsley

Hot pepper sauce

Lemon wedges

INSTRUCTIONS

In a large saucepan combine vegetable broth, 1 teaspoon of the garlic, and 41/2 cups water. Bring to boiling. Gradually stir in grits. Reduce heat. Cook, uncovered, 40 to 50 minutes or until thickened and grits are tender, stirring frequently.

For hash, in an extra-large skillet cook onion, bell pepper, celery, carrots, and the remaining garlic over medium 5 minutes, stirring occasionally and adding water, 1 to 2 tablespoons at a time, as needed to prevent sticking. Add Cajun seasoning; cook and stir 1 minute. Add tomatoes, red beans, and green beans. Cook 5 to 7 minutes or until tomatoes start to break down and green beans are tender, adding water as needed. Season with salt and black pepper.

Serve hash over grits. Sprinkle with parsley and serve with hot sauce and lemon wedges.

Vegan Chilaquiles

INGREDIENTS

3 6-inch corn tortillas, cut into wedges

1 14.5-oz. can no-salt-added fire-roasted diced tomatoes

11/2 cups low-sodium vegetable broth or water

1/2 cup chopped onion

1 small jalapeño chile, halved and seeded, if desired

2 cloves garlic, halved

1/2 teaspoon salt

3 cups cooked red or tricolor quinoa

1 tablespoon nutritional yeast

1 tablespoon salt-free taco seasoning

1 teaspoon smoked paprika

1 15-oz. can no-salt-added black beans, rinsed and drained (11/2 cups)

1/2 cup sliced scallions

Chopped fresh cilantro

INSTRUCTIONS

Preheat oven to 400°F. Spread tortilla wedges on a baking sheet. Bake 10 to 12 minutes or until toasted.

In a blender combine undrained tomatoes, 1 cup of the broth, the onion, jalapeño, garlic, and salt. Cover and blend until smooth. Transfer to a large nonstick skillet. Cook over medium 8 to 10 minutes or until slightly thickened. Stir in tortilla wedges until coated. Cook 2 minutes or until heated through.

Meanwhile, in a medium saucepan combine quinoa, the remaining 1/2 cup broth, the nutritional yeast, taco seasoning, and smoked paprika. Cook over medium 4 to 5 minutes or until broth is mostly absorbed.

Spoon quinoa mixture into shallow dishes. Top with tortilla mixture, beans, scallions, and cilantro.

Tofu Casserole with Mushrooms and Spinach

INGREDIENTS

2 cups chopped red onion

16 oz. fresh cremini or button mushrooms, chopped

2 medium red bell peppers, cut into 1/2-inch dice

1/4 cup chopped fresh parsley

12 cloves garlic, minced

2 teaspoons dried oregano, crushed

2 teaspoons dried thyme, crushed

1 teaspoon ground turmeric

2 12-oz. package extra-firm tofu, drained and crumbled (5 cups)

2 cups packed fresh spinach or arugula

2 tablespoons lemon juice

1 teaspoon black salt or sea salt

Freshly ground black pepper, to taste

8 slices whole wheat bread

1/2 cup cherry tomatoes, halved

Ketchup

INSTRUCTIONS

In a very large skillet cook the first eight **Ingredients** (through turmeric) over medium-high 7 to 8 minutes or until onion is translucent, stirring occasionally and adding water, 1 to 2 tablespoons at a time, as needed to prevent sticking.

Add crumbled tofu; cook 5 to 6 minutes more or until tofu turns yellow and any remaining liquid is cooked off. Add spinach, lemon juice, and salt. Mix well and season with black pepper. Remove from heat.

Cut three slices of bread into 1/2-inch cubes; stir cubes into scramble. Spoon scramble into a 2-quart rectangular baking dish. Let scramble cool completely. Cover and chill until ready to bake.

When ready to bake and serve, remove casserole from refrigerator. Preheat oven to 350°F. Cut the remaining five slices of bread into quarters and insert them decoratively into scramble. Arrange tomatoes over top. Bake 35 minutes or until scramble is heated through and bread is toasted. Serve warm with ketchup

Breakfast Nachos with Vegan Sour Cream

INGREDIENTS

16 6-inch corn tortillas

3 cups cooked brown rice

2 15-oz. cans black beans, rinsed and drained (3 cups)

2 cups fresh or frozen corn

1 cup chopped onion

1 cup chopped red bell pepper

1 cup chopped fresh poblano chile

1/4 cup chopped fresh cilantro

1/4 cup + 3 tablespoons lemon juice

2 tablespoons taco seasoning

11/2 teaspoons garlic powder

12-oz. package extra-firm tofu, drained

1 tablespoon white wine vinegar

1/2 teaspoon sea salt

1/4 teaspoon yellow mustard

1 16-oz. container store-bought pico de gallo

1 avocado, halved, seeded, peeled, and cut into 1/2-inch dice

INSTRUCTIONS

Preheat oven to 350°F. Line two baking sheets with parchment paper. Cut each tortilla into eight triangles. Spread them in a single layer on prepared baking sheets. Bake 20 minutes or until light brown and crispy, turning halfway through baking time. Cool completely. Store chips in an airtight container until ready to use.

In a large bowl stir together the next 7 **Ingredients** (through cilantro), 1/4 cup lemon juice, the taco seasoning, garlic powder, and a pinch of sea salt. Cover and chill until ready to bake.

For Tofu Sour Cream, in a blender combine tofu, remaining 3 tablespoons lemon juice, the white wine vinegar, 1/2 teaspoon sea salt, and the yellow mustard. Cover and blend until smooth. Refrigerate until ready to serve.

When ready to bake and serve, preheat oven to 350°F. Arrange baked chips in a 3-quart rectangular baking dish. Top with bean mixture;

spread in an even layer over chips. Bake, uncovered, 35 minutes or until heated through. Top with Tofu Sour Cream, pico de gallo, and avocado. Serve warm.

Vegan Cinnamon Bun Muffins

INGREDIENTS

11/2 cups spelt flour

1/2 cup oat flour

21/2 teaspoons ground cinnamon

1/2 teaspoon sea salt

2 teaspoons baking powder

1/2 teaspoon baking soda

1/2 cup plain vegan yogurt

1/2 cup pure maple syrup

1/2 cup unsweetened, unflavored plant-based milk

2 tablespoons raisins

2 teaspoons pure vanilla extract

⅓ cup chopped pitted dates

2 tablespoons pure cane sugar

INSTRUCTIONS

Preheat oven to 350°F. Line twelve 21/2-inch muffin cups with paper liners or use silicone muffin cups. In a large bowl combine flours, 11/2 teaspoons of the cinnamon, and 1/4 teaspoon of the salt. Sift baking powder and baking soda into bowl; mix well.

In a medium bowl stir together the next five ingredients (through vanilla). Add to flour mixture. Stir just until flour is moistened. (Do not overmix.) Spoon into prepared muffin cups.

In a small bowl stir together dates, sugar, and the remaining 1 teaspoons cinnamon and 1/4 teaspoon salt. Rub mixture together with your fingertips until small clumps form. Spoon 1 to 2 teaspoons date mixture over batter in each muffin cup.

Bake 20 minutes or until muffins are set to the touch. Let stand in cups 10 minutes. Remove muffins from cups and cool completely on a wire rack. Sprinkle with any remaining date mixture.

Apple Breakfast Casserole with Cherry Drizzle

INGREDIENTS

3/4 cup chopped pitted fresh or frozen sweet cherries

1/2 cup chopped walnuts

11/2 cups cooked quinoa

11/2 cups chopped pitted dates

1 cup orange juice

1 tablespoon orange zest

2 teaspoons grated fresh ginger

1 teaspoon ground cinnamon

4 Gala or Fuji apples, cored and very thinly sliced

2 tablespoons almond or sesame butter (see tip in intro)

1 tablespoon sesame seeds

INSTRUCTIONS

Set aside 1/4 cup of the cherries and 2 tablespoons of the walnuts to garnish the finished casserole. Store them separately in the refrigerator.

In a medium bowl stir together 1/4 cup of the remaining cherries, the remaining walnuts, the quinoa, 3/4 cup of the dates, 1/2 cup of the orange juice, 11/2 teaspoons of the orange zest, the ginger, and cinnamon.

In a 2-quart rectangular baking dish arrange half of the apple slices in an overlapping pattern so they cover bottom of dish. Spread quinoa mixture evenly over apples. Layer the remaining apples over top. Cover surface of apples with plastic wrap (to prevent browning); refrigerate up to 2 days.

For cherry sauce, in a blender combine the remaining 3/4 cup dates, 1/4 cup cherries, 1/2 cup orange juice, and 11/2 teaspoons zest; the almond butter; and 1/2 cup water. Cover and blend until smooth. Chill until ready to bake.

When ready to bake and serve, remove sauce from refrigerator and let warm to room temperature. Preheat oven to 375°F. Remove plastic wrap from dish and cover with foil. Bake, covered, 35 to 40 minutes or until heated through and apples on top start to soften. Remove from oven and let stand, covered, 5 minutes.

Drizzle sauce over casserole and sprinkle with reserved cherries and walnuts and the sesame seeds. Serve warm.

Sweet Congee with Dates and Apricots

INGREDIENTS

4 cups cooked brown rice

1/2 cup chopped pitted dates

1/2 cup chopped dried apricots

1 large stick cinnamon

1/4 teaspoon ground cloves

Sea salt, to taste

INSTRUCTIONS

In a large saucepan bring 2 cups water to boiling over medium. Stir in the first five **Ingredients** (through cloves). Reduce heat to medium-low.

Cook 15 minutes or until mixture thickens into a porridge. Remove cinnamon stick, season with salt, and serve hot

Morning Bangkok Salad

INGREDIENTS

2 tablespoons reduced-sodium tamari or soy sauce

2 tablespoons lime juice

1 tablespoon grated fresh ginger

2 teaspoons lime zest

Pinch crushed red pepper

Freshly ground black pepper, to taste

2 cups cooked brown rice

2 cups bean sprouts

2 cups shredded napa cabbage

1 cup shredded red cabbage

1 cup sliced Persian cucumber

1/2 cup grated carrot

1/2 cup thinly sliced scallions

1/4 cup roasted peanuts

1/4 cup finely chopped fresh basil (preferably Thai basil)

1/4 cup finely chopped fresh cilantro

2 tablespoons finely chopped shallot

INSTRUCTIONS

For dressing, in a small bowl whisk together the first five **Ingredients** (through crushed red pepper). Whisk in 1/4 cup water. Season with black pepper.

In a large bowl combine the remaining ingredients. Drizzle dressing over salad; toss to combine.

Golden Milk Millet Porridge

INGREDIENTS

2 cups unsweetened, unflavored plant-based milk

1/2 teaspoon grated fresh ginger

1/2 teaspoon ground turmeric

6 tablespoons pure maple syrup or date sugar

3 cups cooked millet

1 apple, cored and chopped (11/2 cups)

⅓ cup chopped dried fruit, such as raisins, currants, and/or apricots

3 tablespoons sliced unsalted almonds

INSTRUCTIONS

For golden milk, in a medium saucepan bring milk to boiling. Add ginger and turmeric; reduce heat. Simmer, uncovered, 2 to 3 minutes or until very fragrant, stirring frequently. Whisk in maple syrup. Strain and discard solids; set milk aside.

Add millet and 1 cup water to saucepan. Cover and cook over medium 10 minutes. Reserve a few pieces of apple and dried fruit for garnish. Stir the remaining apple and dried fruit into the saucepan.

Spoon porridge into serving bowls and top with reserved fruits and the almonds. Drizzle warm golden milk over top.

HALLELUJAH DIET LUNCH RECIPES

Rainbow Grain Bowl with Cashew Sauce

Ingredients

3/4 cup unsalted cashews

1/2 cup water

1/4 cup packed parsley leaves

1 tablespoon lemon juice or cider vinegar

1 tablespoon extra-virgin olive oil

1/2 teaspoon reduced-sodium tamari or soy sauce
(see Tip)

1/4 teaspoon salt

1/2 cup cooked lentils

1/2 cup cooked quinoa

1/2 cup shredded red cabbage

1/4 cup grated raw beet

1/4 cup chopped bell pepper

1/4 cup grated carrot

1/4 cup sliced cucumber

1 tablespoon Toasted chopped cashews for garnish

INSTRUCTIONS

Blend cashews, water, parsley, lemon juice (or vinegar), oil, tamari (or soy sauce) and salt in a blender until smooth.

Place lentils and quinoa in the center of a shallow serving bowl. Top with cabbage, beet, pepper, carrot and cucumber. Spoon 2 tablespoons of the cashew sauce over the top (save extra sauce for another use). Garnish with cashews, if desired.

Avocado & White Bean Wrap

Ingredients

2 tablespoons cider vinegar

1 tablespoon canola oil

2 teaspoons finely chopped canned chipotle chile in adobo sauce, (see Note)

1/4 teaspoon salt

2 cups shredded red cabbage

1 medium carrot, shredded

1/4 cup chopped fresh cilantro

1 15-ounce can white beans, rinsed

1 ripe avocado

1/2 cup shredded sharp Cheddar cheese

2 tablespoons minced red onion

4 8- to 10-inch whole-wheat wraps, or tortillas

INSTRUCTIONS

Whisk vinegar, oil, chipotle chile and salt in a medium bowl. Add cabbage, carrot and cilantro; toss to combine.

Mash beans and avocado in another medium bowl with a potato masher or fork. Stir in cheese and onion.

To assemble the wraps, spread about 1/2 cup of the bean-avocado mixture onto a wrap (or tortilla) and top with about 2/3 cup of the cabbage-carrot slaw.

Roll up. Repeat with remaining **Ingredients**. Cut the wraps in half to serve, if desired.

Tomato-&-Avocado Cheese Sandwich

Ingredients

2 slices whole-wheat bread

1/4 avocado, mashed

3 slices tomato

1/4 cup grated Parmesan cheese

1 cup mixed salad greens or baby spinach

2 teaspoons balsamic vinegar

1 medium ripe pear

INSTRUCTIONS

Lay bread on work surface. Spread avocado on one slice. Top with tomatoes and sprinkle with cheese. Toast both pieces of bread in a toaster oven until the plain piece is toasted and the cheese is starting to melt on the topped piece, 4 to 6 minutes.

Remove the toast from the toaster oven with a spatula, and mound greens (or spinach) on top of the cheese side. Drizzle with vinegar and top with the remaining toast. Cut in half if desired and serve with pear.

Roasted Veggie Mason Jar Salad

Ingredients

2 tablespoons Creamy Vegan Cashew Sauce (see associated recipes)

1 cup roasted tofu (see associated recipes)

1 tablespoon pumpkin seeds

1 cup roasted vegetables (see associated recipes)

2 cups mixed greens

INSTRUCTIONS

Layer into a 4-cup jar, in this order: sauce, tofu, pumpkin seeds, veggies and greens. Close tightly and refrigerate for up to 5 days

Turmeric Rice Bowl with Garam Masala Root

Ingredients

Rice

1 1/4 cups water

1/2 cup brown basmati rice

1/4 cup raisins

1 teaspoon extra-virgin olive oil

1 teaspoon onion powder or garlic powder

1/2 teaspoon ground turmeric or 1 teaspoon freshly grated turmeric

1/4 teaspoon ground cinnamon

1/4 teaspoon ground black pepper

1/8 teaspoon kosher salt

Vegetables & Chickpeas

2 tablespoons coconut oil or ghee

1 (15 ounce) can chickpeas, rinsed and patted dry

1 teaspoon garam masala or Indian curry powder

1 cup roasted root vegetables (see associated recipe)

1 teaspoon sugar or honey

1/4 teaspoon kosher salt

1/4 teaspoon ground pepper

2 tablespoons lemon juice

2 tablespoons low-fat plain yogurt or tahini

Chopped fresh herbs, such as mint, parsley and/or cilantro, for garnish

INSTRUCTIONS

To prepare rice: Combine water, rice, raisins, olive oil, onion powder (or garlic powder), turmeric, cinnamon, pepper and 1/8 teaspoon salt in a small saucepan. Bring to a boil. Cover, reduce heat to maintain a gentle simmer and cook until the liquid is absorbed, 35 to 40 minutes. Remove from heat and let stand, covered, for 10 minutes.

Meanwhile, to prepare vegetables & chickpeas: Heat coconut oil (or ghee) in a medium skillet over medium heat. Add chickpeas and cook, stirring, until crispy, 3 to 5 minutes. Stir in garam masala (or curry powder) and cook until fragrant, about 1 minute. Add roasted root vegetables, sugar (or honey), salt and pepper; cook, stirring often, until heated through, 2 to 4 minutes. Stir in lemon juice.

Serve the vegetable mixture over the rice, topped with yogurt (or tahini). Garnish with herbs, if desired.

Chickpea Pasta with Lemony-Parsley Pesto

Ingredients

4 ounces chickpea penne or other penne pasta (about 1 1/4 cups dry)

1 bunch flat-leaf parsley (about 4 cups lightly packed), plus more for garnish

3 cloves garlic

⅓ cup extra-virgin olive oil

1 teaspoon lemon zest

2 tablespoons lemon juice

1/2 teaspoon kosher salt

1/4 teaspoon ground black pepper

1 1/2 cups roasted root vegetables (see associated recipe)

INSTRUCTIONS

Cook pasta according to package directions. Drain well.

Meanwhile, combine parsley and garlic in a food processor and pulse until uniformly chopped, about 10 times. Add oil, lemon juice, salt and pepper and puree until just combined, about 15 seconds; it should be chunky.

Microwave roasted root vegetables in a microwave-safe bowl until heated through, about 1 minute. (Alternatively, heat 1 teaspoon extra-virgin olive oil in a large skillet over medium-high heat. Add vegetables and cook, stirring often, until heated through, 2 to 4 minutes.)

Toss the hot pasta with the pesto, the vegetables and lemon zest. Garnish with parsley, if desired.

Vegetarian Italian Hoagies

Ingredients

1/4 cup thinly sliced red onion, separated into rings

1 14-ounce can artichoke hearts, rinsed and coarsely chopped

1 medium tomato, seeded and diced

2 tablespoons balsamic vinegar

1 tablespoon extra-virgin olive oil

1 teaspoon dried oregano

1 16- to 20-inch-long baguette, preferably whole-grain

2 slices provolone cheese, (about 2 ounces), halved

2 cups shredded romaine lettuce

1/4 cup sliced pepperoncini, (optional)

INSTRUCTIONS

Place onion rings in a small bowl and add cold water to cover. Set aside while you prepare the remaining ingredients.

Combine artichoke hearts, tomato, vinegar, oil and oregano in a medium bowl. Cut baguette into 4 equal lengths. Split each piece horizontally and pull out about half of the soft bread from each side. Drain the onions and pat dry.

To assemble sandwiches, divide provolone among the bottom pieces of baguette. Spread on the artichoke mixture and top with the onion, lettuce and pepperoncini, if using. Cover with the baguette tops. Serve immediately.

Tomato & Provolone Sandwiches

Ingredients

1 small clove garlic, finely chopped

1/4 cup low-fat mayonnaise

2 tablespoons chopped fresh tarragon or basil or 1 teaspoon dried

1 tablespoon lemon juice

1/4 teaspoon freshly ground pepper

Pinch of salt

8 slices whole-grain country bread

4 slices provolone cheese (about 4 ounces)

2 large or 3 medium tomatoes (about 1 1/2 pounds), sliced 1/2 inch thick

INSTRUCTIONS

Position rack in upper third of oven; preheat broiler.

Mash garlic on a cutting board with the side of a chef's knife or a spoon until a paste forms. Transfer to a small bowl and combine with mayonnaise, tarragon (or basil), lemon juice, pepper and salt.

Place bread on a large baking sheet and broil until lightly toasted, 1 to 2 minutes. Turn the bread over and divide cheese among 4 of the pieces. Continue broiling until the cheese is melted, 1 to 2 minutes.

Assemble sandwiches with tomato and the garlic-herb mayonnaise. Top with the melted cheese bread.

Black Bean-Avocado Torta

Ingredients

1 15-ounce can black beans, or pinto beans, rinsed (see Note)

3 tablespoons prepared salsa

1 tablespoon chopped pickled jalapeño

1/2 teaspoon ground cumin

1 ripe avocado, pitted

2 tablespoons minced onion

1 tablespoon lime juice

1 16- to 20-inch-long baguette, preferably whole-grain

1 ⅓ cups shredded green cabbage

INSTRUCTIONS

Mash beans, salsa, jalapeno and cumin in a small bowl. Mash avocado, onion and lime juice in another small bowl.

Cut baguette into 4 equal lengths. Split each piece in half horizontally. Pull out most of the soft bread from the center so you're left with mostly crust. Divide the bean paste, avocado mixture and cabbage evenly among the sandwiches. Cut each in half and serve.

Note

While we love the convenience of canned beans, they tend to be high in sodium. Give them a good rinse before adding to a recipe to rid them of some of their sodium (up to 35 percent) or opt for low-sodium or no-salt-added varieties. (This recipe is analyzed with rinsed, regular canned beans.) Or, if you have the time, cook your own beans from scratch.

Layered Black Rice Salad

INGREDIENTS

2 tablespoons rice vinegar

2 tablespoons lime juice

2 tablespoons reduced-sodium soy sauce

2 teaspoons pure maple syrup

1 teaspoons sriracha sauce

1/2 teaspoon red pepper flakes

4 cups cooled cooked black rice

2 cups fresh or thawed frozen edamame

2 cups shredded carrots

1 medium red bell pepper, cut into thin strips

1/2 cup thinly sliced halved red onion

1 cup coarsely chopped fresh herbs, such as mint, Thai basil, and/or cilantro

2 tablespoons sesame seeds, toasted

Lime wedges

INSTRUCTIONS

For Spicy Soy Vinaigrette, in a small bowl whisk together brown rice vinegar, lime juice, reduced-sodium soy sauce, maple syrup, sriracha sauce, crushed red pepper, and 2 tablespoons water. Dressing can be refrigerated until ready to serve.

In a large glass bowl, layer half each of the rice, edamame, carrots, bell pepper, onion, fresh herbs, Spicy Soy Vinaigrette, and sesame seeds. Repeat layers. Serve with lime wedges and garnish with additional fresh herbs.

Kale and Lentil Salad with Potatoes

INGREDIENTS

2 tablespoons lemon juice

1 teaspoon yellow mustard

1/2 teaspoon garlic powder

1/2 teaspoon paprika

1/8 teaspoon freshly ground black pepper

4 cups thinly sliced kale leaves, stems removed

1 cup dry brown lentils, rinsed and drained

1 lb. Yukon gold potatoes, cut into 3/4-inch dice (3 cups)

1/2 cup shredded carrot

Sea salt, to taste

INSTRUCTIONS

For dressing, in a large bowl whisk together the first five **Ingredients** (through pepper) and 2 tablespoons water. Add kale; toss to coat. Let stand at least 30 minutes.

Meanwhile, in a medium saucepan combine lentils and 3 cups water. Let lentils soak 20 minutes. Bring water to boiling; reduce heat. Cover and simmer 10 minutes or until lentils are tender. Drain any liquid remaining in pan. Let lentils cool at least 10 minutes.

Place potatoes in a steamer basket in a large saucepan. Add water to saucepan to just below basket. Bring to boiling. Steam, covered, 15 minutes or until tender. Transfer potatoes to a large bowl and let cool.

Add cooled lentils and potatoes to bowl with kale. Add carrot; toss to combine. Season with salt. Serve at room temperature or chilled.

Vegan Pineapple Coleslaw

INGREDIENTS

6 cups shredded red and/or green cabbage

1 cup chopped fresh or canned juice-pack pineapple

1/2 cup shredded carrot

1/2 of a 12-oz. package light silken tofu

2 tablespoons lemon juice

1 teaspoon pure cane sugar

1/8 teaspoon cayenne pepper

⅓ to 1/2 cup pineapple juice

Fresh parsley (optional)

INSTRUCTIONS

In a large bowl toss together cabbage, pineapple, and carrot. For dressing, in a small blender or food processor combine tofu, lemon juice, sugar, and cayenne pepper. Cover and blend until smooth, gradually adding pineapple juice until dressing has thick syrup-like consistency.

Drizzle dressing over cabbage mixture; toss to coat. If desired, sprinkle with parsley.

Tabbouleh Salad with Watermelon Radish

INGREDIENTS

2 rounds whole wheat pita bread, cut into wedges

41/2 cups cooked bulgur

4 cups coarsely chopped fresh spinach

1 15-oz. can no-salt-added navy beans, rinsed and drained (11/2 cups)

8 oz. fresh asparagus, trimmed and cut into 1-inch pieces

1 cup chopped fresh parsley

1 cup shredded carrots

1/2 cup sliced watermelon radishes

3 tablespoons lemon juice

2 tablespoons white wine vinegar

2 tablespoons tahini

1 teaspoon pure maple syrup (optional)

1 clove garlic, minced

Sea salt, to taste

Freshly ground black pepper, to taste

Lemon wedges

INSTRUCTIONS

Preheat oven to 375°F. On a baking sheet arrange pita bread wedges in a single layer. Bake 8 to 10 minutes or until lightly browned and crisp. Cool on a wire rack.

In a large bowl toss together the next seven ingredients (through radishes). In a small bowl whisk together the next five ingredients (through garlic) and 1/4 cup water. Add to salad mixture and stir to coat. Season with salt and pepper. Serve with pita and lemon wedges.

Bulgur-Bean Salad with Tomato Vinaigrette

INGREDIENTS

⅔ cup low-sodium tomato juice

3 tablespoons sherry vinegar

2 tablespoons pure maple syrup

1 teaspoon dry mustard

1/2 teaspoon sea salt

1/4 teaspoon cayenne pepper

4 cups cooled cooked bulgur

2 15-oz. cans no-salt-added chickpeas, rinsed and drained (3 cups)

1 15-oz. can no-salt-added small red beans, rinsed and drained (11/2 cups)

1 cup thinly sliced celery

1 cup chopped fresh parsley

1/2 cup finely chopped sweet onion

Baby romaine

Quartered cherry tomatoes

Freshly ground black pepper

INSTRUCTIONS

In a large bowl whisk together the first six **Ingredients** (through cayenne). Add the next six

Ingredients (through onion); toss to coat. Arrange romaine on a serving platter. Spoon bulgur mixture over top. Top with tomatoes and sprinkle with black pepper.

Quinoa Tabbouleh with Pomegranate Seeds

INGREDIENTS

4 cups fresh parsley leaves (about 2 bunches)

2 cups cooked quinoa

1 cup cherry tomatoes, halved

1 Persian cucumber, cut into 1/2-inch dice (1 cup)

1 cup pomegranate arils

1 cup thinly sliced scallions

3 tablespoons lemon juice

Sea salt, to taste

Freshly ground black pepper, to taste

INSTRUCTIONS

In a food processor pulse parsley to the size of rice grains.

In a medium bowl stir together parsley and the remaining **Ingredients**. Taste and adjust seasoning. Serve at room temperature or chilled.

Chopped Salad with Air-Fried BBQ Chickpeas

INGREDIENTS

1 tablespoon + 1/8 teaspoon paprika

11/2 teaspoons ground cumin

1 teaspoon packed brown sugar

11/2 teaspoons garlic powder

11/2 teaspoons onion powder

11/4 teaspoons dry mustard

1/2 teaspoon freshly ground black pepper, plus more for garnish

1/4 teaspoon cayenne pepper

1/4 teaspoon ground cinnamon

11/2 15-oz. cans no-salt-added chickpeas, rinsed and drained (21/4 cups)

2 tablespoons lime juice

6 cups chopped romaine lettuce

2 cups cherry tomatoes, halved

1 cup fresh sweet corn kernels (from 2 ears)

2 cups cooled cooked tricolor quinoa

1/2 cup chopped red bell pepper

1/4 cup chopped red onion

1 avocado, halved, seeded, and peeled

2 tablespoons chopped fresh parsley

⅓ to 1/2 cup unsweetened, unflavored plant-based milk

Sea salt, to taste

Freshly ground black pepper, to taste

INSTRUCTIONS

To make BBQ Spice Blend, stir together 1 tablespoon paprika, 1 teaspoon garlic powder, 1 teaspoon onion powder, and 1 teaspoon dry mustard, 1/2 teaspoon freshly ground black pepper, the cumin, brown sugar, cayenne pepper, and cinnamon in a small bowl. Store in an airtight container. Makes about 3 tablespoons.

For BBQ chickpeas, preheat an air fryer to 360°F. In a medium bowl toss together chickpeas, 1 tablespoon of BBQ Spice Blend, and 1 tablespoon lime juice. Place half in air fryer. Air-fry 10 to 15 minutes or until browned and crisp, stirring occasionally. Transfer to a rimmed baking sheet to cool. Repeat with remaining chickpeas.

In a bowl combine romaine lettuce and the next five ingredients (through red onion). In a blender combine the remaining 1 tablespoon lime juice, the avocado, parsley, remaining 1/2 teaspoon each of garlic powder, onion powder, and dry mustard, and remaining 1/8 teaspoon paprika. Cover and blend until smooth, gradually adding milk to reach drizzling consistency. Drizzle over salad;

toss to coat. Season salad with salt and black pepper. Top with chickpeas.

Hasselback Roasted Zucchini

INGREDIENTS

4 medium zucchini and/or yellow summer squash (8 to 10 oz. each)

2 cups fresh parsley and/or basil leaves

2 teaspoons capers, rinsed and drained

1 teaspoon lemon zest

3 cloves garlic, minced

Sea salt, to taste

1/4 teaspoon freshly ground black pepper

11/2 cups cooked whole wheat couscous, cooled (see tip in intro)

1/4 cup nutritional yeast

2 tablespoons tahini

3 tablespoons lemon juice

INSTRUCTIONS

Preheat oven to 400°F. Line a 15×10-inch baking pan with parchment paper. If necessary, remove a thin slice from one side of each zucchini so it sits flat. Cut each in half crosswise. On a cutting board arrange two chopsticks or wooden spoons lengthwise on either side of zucchini. Cut zucchini crosswise into 1/4-inch slices, stopping when knife reaches chopsticks (to prevent slicing all the way through). Arrange zucchini in prepared pan.

In a food processor combine basil and/or parsley; capers; lemon zest; 2 cloves of the garlic, minced; the sea salt; and black pepper. Pulse until chopped and well combined. Transfer to a medium bowl. Stir in couscous and nutritional yeast. Spoon mixture between slices of zucchini. Spoon any remaining filling over or around zucchini. Roast, uncovered, 25 minutes or until lightly browned and tender.

For Tahini Sauce, in a small food processor combine tahini, lemon juice, and remaining garlic. Process until smooth, gradually adding 2 to 4 tablespoons of water until drizzling consistency.

Serve zucchini drizzled with Tahini Sauce.

Salad with Creamy Pesto Dressing

INGREDIENTS

1/2 cup soaked raw cashews (see tip in recipe intro)

⅔ cup loosely packed fresh basil leaves

1 clove garlic

1 tablespoon nutritional yeast

1/4 teaspoon onion powder

1/4 teaspoon sea salt

⅔ cup unsweetened, unflavored plant-based milk

6 cups fresh baby spinach

4 cups cooled cooked wheat berries

2 cups cherry tomatoes, halved

1 medium summer squash, quartered lengthwise and cut into 1/2- inch slices

1 cup shredded carrots

1/2 cup chopped red onion

Sea salt, to taste

Freshly ground black pepper, to taste

INSTRUCTIONS

For Pesto Dressing, in a small blender or food processor combine the first six **Ingredients** (through sea salt). Cover and blend until smooth, gradually adding plant-based milk. Dressing will be thin.

In four 1-quart wide-mouth Mason jars, pour a few tablespoons of dressing into the bottom. Then layer the next seven **Ingredients** (spinach through onion) in the order given. Season with salt and pepper.

Vegan Grain Bowl

Ingredients

1 medium sweet potato, peeled if desired, cut into 1-inch chunks

3 tablespoons extra-virgin olive oil, divided

1/2 teaspoon salt, divided

1/2 teaspoon ground pepper, divided

2 tablespoons tahini

2 tablespoons water

1 tablespoon lemon juice

1 small clove garlic, minced

2 cups cooked quinoa

1 15-ounce can chickpeas, rinsed

1 firm ripe avocado, diced

1/4 cup chopped fresh cilantro or parsley

INSTRUCTIONS

Preheat oven to 425 degrees F.

Toss sweet potato with 1 tablespoon oil and 1/4 teaspoon each salt and pepper in a medium bowl. Transfer to a rimmed baking sheet. Roast, stirring once, until tender, 15 to 18 minutes.

Meanwhile, whisk the remaining 2 tablespoons oil, tahini, water, lemon juice, garlic and the remaining 1/4 teaspoon each salt and pepper in a small bowl.

To serve, divide quinoa among 4 bowls. Top with equal amounts of sweet potato, chickpeas and avocado. Drizzle with the tahini sauce. Sprinkle with parsley (or cilantro).

Chicken & Apple Kale Wraps

Ingredients

1 tablespoon mayonnaise

1 teaspoon Dijon mustard

3 medium lacinato kale leaves

3 ounces thinly sliced cooked chicken breast

6 thin red onion slices

1 firm apple, cut into 9 slices

INSTRUCTIONS

Mix mayonnaise and mustard together in a small bowl. Spread on kale leaves. Top each leaf with 1 ounce chicken, 2 slices onion and 3 slices apple. Roll each leaf into a wrap. Cut in half, if desired.

HALLELUJAH DIET RECIPES FOR DINNER

Chile-Lime Cauliflower Quesadillas

Ingredients

3 tablespoons corn oil, divided

1 tablespoon tablespoon chili-lime seasoning or rub, such as Tajín (see Tip)

2 cups chopped cauliflower

1 cup chopped poblano peppers

8 (6 inch) corn or whole-wheat tortillas, warmed

1/2 cup reduced-sodium refried black beans

3/4 cup shredded Cheddar cheese

Salsa for serving

INSTRUCTIONS

Position rack in upper third of oven; preheat broiler to high. Line a baking sheet with foil.

Whisk 1 tablespoon oil and seasoning in a medium bowl. Add cauliflower and poblanos; toss to coat. Spread evenly on the prepared pan. Broil on the upper rack until just tender, about 8 minutes. Reduce oven temperature to 200 degrees .

Top half of each tortilla with 1 tablespoon each beans and cheese and 1/4 cup of the vegetable mixture. Sprinkle with the remaining cheese. Fold the tortillas in half.

Heat 1 tablespoon oil in a large nonstick skillet over medium-high heat. Add 4 quesadillas and cook, flipping once halfway, until browned, 2 to 4 minutes per side. Transfer to the baking sheet and keep warm in the oven. Repeat with the remaining 1 tablespoon oil and 4 quesadillas. Serve the quesadillas with salsa, if desired.

Gochujang-Glazed Tempeh & Brown Rice Bowls

Ingredients

1/2 cup water, divided

5 tablespoons rice vinegar, divided

4 tablespoons reduced-sodium tamari, divided

4 tablespoons light brown sugar, divided

2 cups thinly sliced napa cabbage

1 cup thinly sliced radishes

1 tablespoon gochujang

3 cloves garlic, minced

1 teaspoon grated peeled fresh ginger

1 tablespoon cornstarch

8 ounces tempeh, cut crosswise into 16 pieces

2 cups cooked brown rice

1/4 cup fresh cilantro

INSTRUCTIONS

Preheat oven to 425 degrees F. Set a wire rack on a rimmed baking sheet and coat with cooking spray.

Whisk 1/4 cup water, 4 tablespoons vinegar and 1 tablespoon each tamari and brown sugar in a medium bowl. Add cabbage and radishes and toss to combine. Set aside, tossing occasionally.

Meanwhile, combine the remaining 1 tablespoon vinegar, 3 tablespoons each tamari and brown sugar, gochujang, garlic and ginger in a small saucepan. Bring to a simmer over medium-high heat. Cook, stirring occasionally, for 2 minutes. Whisk the remaining 1/4 cup water and cornstarch in a small bowl. Slowly add the cornstarch mixture to the sauce, whisking constantly. Cook until thickened, about 1 minute.

Pour half the sauce into a medium bowl and add tempeh; gently toss to coat. Transfer the tempeh to the prepared rack. Bake until the sauce is tacky, about 15 minutes. Return the tempeh to the bowl and add the remaining sauce. Gently toss to coat.

Divide rice among 4 bowls. Transfer the pickled vegetables to the bowls using a slotted spoon;

drizzle with the liquid, if desired. Top with the tempeh and sprinkle with cilantro.

Asparagus & Purple Artichoke Pizza

Ingredients

1 tablespoon cornmeal

1 pound whole-wheat pizza dough, at room temperature

2 tablespoons extra-virgin olive oil, divided

2 cloves garlic, sliced

1/4 teaspoon kosher salt, divided

1/8 teaspoon crushed red pepper

1 1/2 cups shredded part-skim mozzarella cheese

2 baby purple artichokes

1 teaspoon lemon zest

2 tablespoons lemon juice

8 ounces purple asparagus, trimmed

2 ounces shaved pecorino cheese (1/2 cup)

1/4 teaspoon ground pepper

Purple shiso leaves for serving

INSTRUCTIONS

Position rack in lower third of oven; preheat to 450 degrees F. Sprinkle a baking sheet with cornmeal.

Roll out dough on a lightly floured surface into a 12-inch oval. Transfer to the prepared pan and brush with 1 tablespoon oil. Sprinkle the dough with garlic, 1/8 teaspoon salt and crushed red pepper, then top with mozzarella. Bake until bubbling and golden brown, 12 to 15 minutes.

Meanwhile, snap the tough outer leaves off artichokes and cut off the top two-thirds, down to the heart. Peel the tough stem. Cut the artichokes in half and remove any fuzzy choke. Thinly slice the artichokes and toss in a bowl with lemon juice. Shave asparagus into long strips using a vegetable peeler; thinly slice what can't be shaved. Add the asparagus to the bowl along with pecorino, pepper, the remaining 1 tablespoon oil and 1/8 teaspoon salt; toss to coat.

Top the pizza with the vegetables and sprinkle with lemon zest and shiso, if using.

Spring Veggie Wraps

Ingredients

1 (14 ounce) package package extra-firm tofu, drained and cut into 1/4-inch-thick planks

1/4 cup tahini

1/4 cup orange juice plus 2 Tbsp., divided

1 tablespoon lime juice

1 tablespoon low-sodium soy sauce

1 tablespoon minced fresh ginger

1 clove garlic, minced

2 teaspoons canola or avocado oil, divided

1/4 teaspoon salt, divided

8 large leaves butter, Boston, or Bibb lettuce

1 cup shredded carrot

6 medium radishes, thinly sliced

2 tablespoons thinly sliced scallions (white and light green parts only)

4 8-inch spinach or whole-wheat tortillas, warmed

2 tablespoons black or white sesame seeds

INSTRUCTIONS

Line a large baking sheet with 3 layers of paper towels. Arrange tofu in a single layer on it. Cover with another 2 layers of paper towels. Gently press on the tofu to remove excess liquid. Transfer the tofu to a 9x13-inch baking dish.

Whisk tahini, 1/4 cup orange juice, lime juice, soy sauce, ginger, and garlic in a small bowl. Refrigerate 1/4 cup of the mixture to use as sauce. Whisk the remaining 2 Tbsp. orange juice into the mixture in the bowl. Pour the marinade over the tofu and turn to coat. Cover and refrigerate for 30 minutes, turning once or twice.

Discard any unabsorbed marinade. Heat 1 tsp. oil in a large nonstick skillet over medium-high heat. Reduce heat to medium. Add half the tofu; sprinkle with 1/8 tsp. salt. Cook for 5 minutes. Flip and cook until lightly browned, 4 to 6 minutes more. Adjust heat as necessary to prevent burning. Transfer the tofu to a plate and keep warm. Repeat with the remaining 1 tsp. oil, tofu, and the remaining 1/8 tsp. salt.

Divide lettuce, carrot, radishes, and scallions among tortillas, arranging the vegetables down the center of each tortilla. Top with tofu and drizzle with the reserved tahini sauce. Sprinkle with sesame seeds, then roll up

Mushroom Pizzas with Arugula Salad

Ingredients

8 large portobello mushroom caps (about 4 oz. each), gills removed (see Tip)

2 tablespoons olive oil plus 1 tsp., divided

1/2 teaspoon ground pepper, divided

1/2 cup pizza or tomato sauce

2 cups lightly packed baby spinach, chopped

1/2 cup sun-dried tomatoes (about 8), chopped

1 (14 ounce) can artichoke hearts, rinsed and chopped

1/2 cup shredded part-skim mozzarella cheese

1/4 cup crumbled feta cheese

1/2 teaspoon dried Italian seasoning

1 tablespoon lemon juice

2 cups lightly packed baby arugula

1/4 cup fresh basil leaves, thinly sliced

INSTRUCTIONS

Preheat oven to 400 degrees F. Line a large baking sheet with foil and set a wire rack on it. Brush tops of portobello caps with 1 Tbsp. oil and place them, undersides-up, on the rack. Roast for 10 minutes. Flip and roast for 5 minutes more.

Remove the portobellos from the oven and carefully flip them back over so that the undersides are up. Season with 1/4 tsp. pepper. Spread 1 Tbsp. sauce inside each cap. Divide spinach, sun-dried tomatoes, artichokes, mozzarella, and feta among the caps. Sprinkle with Italian seasoning. Return the portobellos to the oven and bake until the cheese is melted and starting to brown, 10 to 15 minutes.

Meanwhile, whisk the remaining 1 Tbsp. plus 1 tsp. oil, the remaining 1/8 tsp. pepper, and lemon juice in a medium bowl. Add arugula and toss to coat.

Garnish the portobello pizzas with basil and serve with the arugula salad.

Spinach Ravioli with Artichokes & Olives

Ingredients

2 (8 ounce) packages frozen or refrigerated spinach-and-ricotta ravioli

1/2 cup oil-packed sun-dried tomatoes, drained (2 tablespoons oil reserved)

1 (10 ounce) package frozen quartered artichoke hearts, thawed

1 (15 ounce) can no-salt-added cannellini beans, rinsed

1/4 cup Kalamata olives, sliced

3 tablespoons toasted pine nuts

1/4 cup chopped fresh basil

INSTRUCTIONS

Bring a large pot of water to a boil. Cook ravioli according to package directions. Drain and toss with 1 tablespoon reserved oil; set aside.

Heat the remaining 1 tablespoon oil in a large nonstick skillet over medium heat. Add artichokes and beans; sauté until heated through, 2 to 3 minutes.

Fold in the cooked ravioli, sun-dried tomatoes, olives, pine nuts and basil.

Vegetarian Lettuce Wraps

Ingredients

3 tablespoons rice vinegar

2 tablespoons hoisin sauce

2 tablespoons reduced-sodium soy sauce

1 teaspoon sesame oil

1/4 teaspoon crushed red pepper

1 (14 ounce) package extra-firm tofu

1 tablespoon canola oil

8 ounces white mushrooms, finely chopped

1 cup finely chopped daikon radish

3 large cloves garlic, minced

1 tablespoon grated fresh ginger

4 scallions, sliced

8 large leaves Bibb or iceberg lettuce

1/4 cup Julienned carrots

INSTRUCTIONS

Combine vinegar, hoisin, soy sauce, sesame oil and crushed red pepper in a small bowl; set aside.

Cut tofu in half horizontally. Press the tofu slices between paper towels to squeeze out as much liquid as possible. Crumble the tofu. Heat canola oil in a large nonstick skillet over medium-high heat. Add the crumbled tofu; cook, stirring and breaking into smaller pieces, until starting to brown, about 5 minutes. Add mushrooms; continue cooking and stirring until any liquid has evaporated, about 3 minutes. Stir in daikon, garlic, ginger and scallions. Add the reserved sauce; cook, stirring, until well combined and heated through, about 2 minutes.

Spoon a scant 1/2 cup tofu mixture into each lettuce leaf. Top with carrots, if desired.

Gluten-Free Cream of Mushroom Soup

Ingredients

4 tablespoons extra-virgin olive oil, divided

1 cup diced shallots

1/2 cup diced celery

5 cups sliced shiitake mushroom caps (about 10 ounces), divided

5 cups sliced baby bella mushrooms (about 10 ounces), divided

1/2 cup dry sherry

3 cloves garlic, minced

4 cups diced peeled Yukon Gold potatoes (about 1 pound)

1/2 teaspoon dried thyme

3 cups "no-chicken broth" or mushroom broth

1 cup water

1/2 cup walnuts, finely chopped

Pinch of salt

2 teaspoons sherry vinegar

1/2 teaspoon ground pepper

2 tablespoons sliced fresh chives

INSTRUCTIONS

Heat 3 tablespoons oil in a large pot over medium heat. Add shallots and celery; cook, stirring occasionally, until tender, about 3 minutes. Add 4 cups each shiitakes and baby bellas, sherry and garlic; cook, stirring occasionally, until the mushrooms are soft and the liquid has evaporated, about 5 minutes. Stir in potatoes and thyme; cook for 1 minute. Add broth and water. Bring to a boil. Reduce heat to maintain a simmer and cook, stirring occasionally, until the vegetables are very soft, about 20 minutes.

Meanwhile, coarsely chop the remaining 2 cups mushrooms. Heat the remaining 1 tablespoon oil in a medium skillet over medium heat. Add the mushrooms and cook, stirring often, until soft, about 2 minutes. Add walnuts and salt. Cook, stirring occasionally, until hot, about 1 minute more.

Puree the soup with an immersion blender or in a regular blender (in batches, if necessary) until very smooth. (Use caution when blending hot liquids.) Stir in vinegar and pepper.

Serve the soup topped with the mushroom-walnut mixture and chives.

Vegetarian Stuffed Cabbage

Ingredients

1 cup water

1/2 cup short-grain brown rice

1 teaspoon extra-virgin olive oil plus 2 tablespoons, divided

1 large Savoy cabbage (2-3 pounds)

1 pound baby bella mushrooms, finely chopped

1 large onion, finely chopped

4 cloves garlic, minced

1/2 teaspoon dried rubbed sage

1/2 teaspoon crumbled dried rosemary

1/2 teaspoon salt, divided

1/4 teaspoon freshly ground pepper plus 1/8 teaspoon, divided

1/2 cup red wine

1/4 cup dried currants

1/3 cup toasted pine nuts (see Tips), chopped

2 tablespoons extra-virgin olive oil, divided

1 small onion, chopped

garlic, minced

1/4 teaspoon salt

1/4 teaspoon freshly ground pepper

1 28-ounce can no-salt-added crushed tomatoes (see Tips)

1/2 cup red wine

INSTRUCTIONS

To prepare cabbage & filling: Combine water, rice and 1 teaspoon oil in a medium saucepan; bring to a boil. Reduce heat to maintain the barest simmer, cover and cook until the water is absorbed and the rice is just tender, 40 to 50 minutes. Transfer to a large bowl and set aside.

Meanwhile, half fill a large pot with water and bring to a boil. Line a baking sheet with a clean kitchen towel and place near the stove.

Using a small, sharp knife, remove the core from the bottom of the cabbage. Add the cabbage to the boiling water and cook for 5 minutes. As the leaves soften, use tongs to gently remove 8 large outer leaves. Transfer the leaves to the baking sheet and pat with more towels to thoroughly dry. Set aside.

Drain the remaining cabbage in a colander for a few minutes. Finely chop enough to get about 3 cups. (Save any remaining cabbage for another use.)

Heat 1 1/2 tablespoons oil in a large skillet over medium-high heat. Add mushrooms, onion, garlic, sage, rosemary and 1/4 teaspoon each salt and pepper; cook, stirring, until the mushrooms have released their juices and the pan is fairly dry, 8 to 10 minutes. Add wine and cook, stirring, until evaporated, about 3 minutes more. Add the mixture to the cooked rice along with currants and pine nuts.

Heat the remaining 1/2 tablespoon oil in the skillet over medium-high. Add the chopped cabbage, the remaining 1/4 teaspoon salt and 1/8 teaspoon pepper; cook, stirring, until the cabbage is wilted and just beginning to brown, 3 to 5 minutes. Add to the rice mixture.

To prepare sauce: Heat 1 tablespoon oil in a large skillet over medium heat. Add onion, garlic, salt and pepper and cook, stirring, until starting to soften, 2 to 4 minutes. Add tomatoes and wine; bring to a simmer and cook until slightly thickened, about 10 minutes.

Preheat oven to 375 degrees F.

To stuff cabbage: Place a reserved cabbage leaf on your work surface; cut out the thick stem in the center, keeping the leaf intact. Place about 3/4 cup filling in the center. Fold both sides over the filling and roll up. Repeat with the remaining 7 leaves and filling.

Spread 1 cup of the tomato sauce in a 9-by-13-inch baking dish. Place the stuffed cabbage rolls, seam side down, on the sauce. Pour the remaining sauce over the rolls and drizzle with the remaining 1 tablespoon oil.

Bake, uncovered, basting twice with the sauce, until hot, about 45 minutes.

Vegetarian Lo Mein with Shiitakes

Ingredients

8 ounces fresh lo mein noodles or fresh or dried linguine pasta

2 teaspoons toasted sesame oil

3 tablespoons reduced-sodium soy sauce

2 teaspoons Sriracha

2 tablespoons vegetable oil, divided

2 tablespoons minced garlic

1 large carrot, halved lengthwise and cut into 1/4-inch-thick half-moon slices (about 1 cup)

4 ounces fresh shiitake mushrooms, stems removed, caps sliced 1/4-inch thick

1 cup thinly sliced celery

2 cups bean sprouts

3 tablespoons finely chopped fresh cilantro

INSTRUCTIONS

Bring a large pot of water to a boil. Cook noodles according to package directions. Drain, rinse with cold water, and shake out excess water until the noodles are completely dry (pat noodles dry if needed). Transfer to a large bowl and toss with sesame oil; set aside. Combine soy sauce and Sriracha in a small bowl; set aside.

Heat a 14-inch flat-bottomed carbon-steel wok (or 12-inch stainless-steel skillet) over high heat until a drop of water vaporizes within 1 to 2 seconds of contact. Swirl in 1 Tbsp. vegetable oil. Add garlic; stir-fry until just fragrant, about 10 seconds. Add carrot, mushrooms, and celery; stir-fry until the celery is bright green and the vegetables have absorbed all the oil, about 1 minute.

Swirl in the remaining 1 Tbsp. vegetable oil. Add bean sprouts, the noodles, and the soy sauce mixture; stir-fry until the noodles are heated through and the vegetables are tender-crisp, 1 to 2 minutes. Add cilantro and toss to combine.

HALLELUJAH DIET RECIPES FOR SALAD AND SIDE DISH

Orange Farro Salad with Pan-Roasted Tomatoes

INGREDIENTS

4 oranges (navel, Cara Cara, and/or blood oranges)

⅓ cup white wine vinegar

1 tablespoon Dijon mustard

1 tablespoon pure maple syrup

1/2 teaspoon sea salt

1/4 teaspoon freshly ground black pepper

4 cups cooled cooked farro

1 15-oz. can no-salt-added cannellini beans, rinsed and drained (11/2 cups)

1/2 cup slivered red onion or sliced scallions

1/2 cup sliced fresh basil

6 cups fresh baby kale

2 cups grape tomatoes

2 tablespoons chopped toasted hazelnuts

INSTRUCTIONS

Remove 1/2 teaspoon zest from one of the oranges. On a cutting board, slice off the tops and bottoms of all oranges. Slice off the skin and bitter pith in small sections from top to bottom following the curve of the fruit. Holding an orange over a bowl to catch juices, remove segments (supremes) by sliding the knife between the membrane and a segment toward the center of the fruit then back out between the other side of the segment and the next membrane. Repeat to remove all supremes from oranges. Squeeze the membranes to remove any additional juice. Drain juice from bowl into a measuring cup (you should have 3 to 4 tablespoons juice).

For dressing, add the orange zest, vinegar, mustard, maple syrup, salt, and pepper to orange juice in measuring cup; whisk to combine.

Add farro, beans, onion, and basil to bowl with orange supremes; drizzle with half of the dressing (about 5 tablespoons). Stir gently to combine. Place kale in a second bowl. Drizzle kale with 1 tablespoon of the remaining dressing. With clean hands, gently massage dressing into kale until kale is glossy and tender.

In an extra-large skillet cook tomatoes over medium-high 4 to 5 minutes or until lightly charred and skins start to burst, stirring occasionally. Add to farro mixture; stir gently to combine.

Arrange kale on a serving platter. Top with farro mixture. Sprinkle with hazelnuts. Serve with remaining dressing.

Cornucopia Kale Salad

INGREDIENTS

41/2 to 5 cups 1-inch cubes orange sweet potatoes

1/4 cup apple cider vinegar

1/4 cup nutritional yeast

11/2 tablespoons pure maple syrup

11/2 tablespoons tahini

1 tablespoon tamari

1 small clove garlic, halved

1/2 teaspoons yellow mustard

1/4 teaspoons sea salt

5 cups stemmed and chopped kale

1/4 cup raw or toasted pepitas or toasted walnut or

pecan pieces

1/4 cup pomegranate arils or 2 to 3 tablespoons

dried cranberries

INSTRUCTIONS

Preheat oven to 425°F. Line a baking sheet with

parchment paper; sprinkle a few pinches of sea salt

over parchment. Spread sweet potato cubes on the

prepared baking sheet. Bake 35 to 40 minutes or until fully tender and browned in spots, stirring two or three times.

For Buddha Dressing, in a blender (or a deep cup if using an immersion blender) combine apple cider vinegar, nutritional yeast, maple syrup, tahini, tamari, garlic, yellow mustard, and 1/4 teaspoon sea salt. Blend until smooth. Taste and adjust seasoning; thin with water if you like. Store in an airtight container in the fridge until ready to use.

In a large bowl combine hot sweet potatoes and the kale. Toss to slightly wilt kale. Add Buddha Dressing; toss to coat, adding more dressing as desired. Top salad with pepitas and pomegranate arils.

Middle Eastern Red Rice Pilaf

INGREDIENTS

1 cup chopped onion

2 cloves garlic, minced

1 teaspoon Aleppo pepper, or 3/4 teaspoon paprika plus 1/4 teaspoon cayenne pepper

3/4 teaspoon sea salt

1/2 teaspoon ground cinnamon

1/4 teaspoon ground cloves

1/4 teaspoon ground cardamom

21/2 cups dry red rice

11/4 cups chopped peeled acorn squash or butternut squash

⅓ cup raisins

1⅓ cups finely chopped cucumber

2 tablespoons chopped fresh mint

1 teaspoon sesame seeds, toasted

INSTRUCTIONS

In a large saucepan cook onion and garlic over medium 4 minutes or until tender, stirring occasionally and adding water, 1 to 2 tablespoons at a time, as needed to prevent sticking. Stir in Aleppo pepper, salt, cinnamon, cloves, and cardamom. Cook 1 minute.

Add rice and squash; stir to coat. Add 31/2 cups water and the raisins. Bring to boiling; reduce heat. Cover and simmer 30 minutes or until liquid is absorbed. Remove from heat; let stand 10 minutes.

For topper, in a small bowl stir together cucumber, mint, and sesame seeds. Serve with rice mixture.

Black Rice, Roasted Beet, and Orange Salad

INGREDIENTS

2 medium beets (12 oz.), peeled and cut into 1-inch pieces

Sea salt, to taste

Freshly ground black pepper, to taste

2 oranges

⅓ cup chopped toasted walnuts

1 tablespoon Dijon mustard

1/2 teaspoon garlic powder

3 cups cooked black rice, chilled

11/2 cups cooked tricolor quinoa, chilled

1 Granny Smith apple, cored and cut into 1-inch pieces

1 shallot, sliced

INSTRUCTIONS

Preheat oven to 375°F. Place beets in a 2-quart baking dish with 2 tablespoons water; season with salt and pepper. Cover dish with foil. Bake 30 minutes. Uncover; bake 15 to 30 minutes more or until tender and edges are lightly browned.

Meanwhile, zest and juice one of the oranges. Cut the second orange into supremes (see tip in intro) and place in a bowl.

In a small food processor combine 1/4 cup of the walnuts, 1/4 cup orange juice, 1 teaspoon orange zest, the mustard, garlic powder, and 2 tablespoons water. Process until smooth. Season with salt and pepper.

Add rice, quinoa, apple, shallot, and dressing to bowl with orange supremes. Toss to combine. Top with beets and the remaining walnuts.

Good Garlicky Mashed Potatoes

INGREDIENTS

6 large Yukon Gold potatoes, unpeeled

1 bunch kale (optional), stems stripped and leaves torn into bite-size pieces

6 tablespoons nutritional yeast flakes

2 to 3 garlic cloves, minced

1 to 2 cups unsweetened, unflavored almond milk or other plant milk of your choice, or water

1 teaspoon dried rosemary

Freshly ground black pepper

INSTRUCTIONS

Cut the potatoes into 1-inch chunks. Place them in a large pot. Add water to cover and bring the water to boiling. Cook until the potatoes are tender, about 10 minutes.

Meanwhile, bring a separate large pot of water to boiling for the kale, if using. Place kale leaves in the water, cover and cook until tender, about 5 minutes. Drain kale and let it cool in the colander. When kale is cool enough to handle, chop 1 or 2 cups of it into bite-size pieces.

Drain potatoes, transfer them to a large bowl, and mash them with a potato masher. Add the nutritional yeast and garlic; then add the almond milk a little at a time, mashing until smooth and creamy. They will need more liquid than you might expect since the nutritional yeast soaks up liquid.

Stir in the rosemary and season with pepper to taste. Gently fold in the kale. Serve warm.

Vegan Waldorf Salad

INGREDIENTS

4 red and green apples, cored and chopped

4 cups cooled cooked barley

3 stalks celery, diagonally sliced

3/4 cup raisins

1/2 of a 12-oz. package soft silken tofu

1/2 cup apple cider or apple juice

2 tablespoons lemon juice

1 tablespoon apple cider vinegar

1 tablespoon pure maple syrup

1/4 teaspoon pumpkin pie spice

Dash cayenne pepper

Sea salt, to taste

Freshly ground black pepper, to taste

Bibb lettuce leaves (optional)

Pumpkin pie spice, chopped fresh parsley, and/or
2 tablespoons chopped walnuts (optional)

INSTRUCTIONS

In a large bowl combine apples, barley, celery, and raisins. In a small food processor or blender combine the next seven ingredients (through cayenne pepper). Process until smooth. Pour over salad and toss to coat. Season with salt and black pepper.

If you like, serve salad in Bibb lettuce leaf cups and sprinkle with pumpkin pie spice, parsley, and/or walnuts.

Plantain Salad with Black Beans and Rice

INGREDIENTS

4 plantains, peeled and cut into 1/2-inch slices

1 large red onion, cut into wedges

⅓ cup orange juice

3 tablespoons lemon juice

3 tablespoons lime juice

1 teaspoon chopped fresh oregano

1 teaspoon ground cumin

1/4 teaspoon sea salt

2 15-oz. cans no-salt-added black beans, rinsed and drained (3 cups)

4 cups thinly sliced kale leaves, stems removed (see tip in intro)

3 cups cherry tomatoes, halved

2 cups cooled cooked brown rice

1 teaspoon coarse ground mustard

1 teaspoon pure maple syrup

Sea salt, to taste

Freshly ground black pepper, to taste

Orange, lemon, and/or lime wedges (optional)

INSTRUCTIONS

Preheat oven to 400°F. Line a 15×10- inch baking pan with parchment paper or a silicone baking mat. Spread plantains and onion in pan. In a small bowl stir together the next six ingredients (through 1/4 teaspoon salt). Brush 2 tablespoons of the mixture over plantains and onion, reserving the remaining juice mixture for dressing. Roast plantains and onion 20 to 25 minutes or until tender. Cool in pan on a wire rack.

In an extra-large bowl combine cooled plantains and onion, the beans, kale, tomatoes, and rice. Whisk mustard and maple syrup into the remaining juice mixture. Season with salt and pepper. Drizzle over salad; toss to coat. Serve with citrus wedges.

Maple-Glazed Carrots with Thyme

INGREDIENTS

3 cups bias-sliced carrots

1/4 cup low-sodium vegetable broth

2 teaspoons chopped fresh thyme

2 teaspoons pure maple syrup

11/2 tablespoons chopped toasted pecans

INSTRUCTIONS

In a large nonstick skillet combine carrots, broth, thyme, and maple syrup. Cover and cook over medium 12 minutes or until carrots are crisp-tender. Uncover; increase heat to medium-high. Cook 3 minutes or until liquid is reduced and carrots are glazed, stirring often. Sprinkle with pecans. If you like, season with freshly ground black pepper.

Rainbow Veggie Salad with Creamy Harissa Dressing

INGREDIENTS

1/2 cup Homemade Harissa

11/2 tablespoons tahini

1 tablespoon lemon juice

Sea salt, to taste

8 cups baby romaine leaves

1 cup shredded carrots

1 cup halved cherry tomatoes

1 cup chopped red bell pepper

1 thinly sliced Persian cucumber

INSTRUCTIONS

In a blender combine the Homemade Harissa, tahini, lemon juice, and 1/2 cup water. Cover and blend until smooth. Season dressing to taste with sea salt.

In a large bowl combine romaine leaves, shredded carrots, cherry tomatoes, red bell pepper, and Persian cucumber. Add half of the dressing; toss to coat. Add more dressing to taste. Serve immediately.

Cardamom Roasted Carrots with Pomegranate Seeds

INGREDIENTS

3 lb. small to medium whole multicolor carrots, trimmed

2 tablespoons lemon juice

2 tablespoons tahini

2 teaspoons ground cardamom

1/2 teaspoon ground cinnamon

1/4 teaspoon cayenne pepper

1/2 cup pomegranate seeds

Freshly ground black pepper, to taste

INSTRUCTIONS

Preheat oven to 400°F. Line a large rimmed baking sheet with parchment paper or a silicone baking mat. Place carrots on prepared baking sheet. In a small bowl whisk together the next five ingredients (through cayenne pepper) and 1/4 cup water. Lightly brush mixture over carrots.

Roast carrots about 40 minutes or until browned and tender, brushing lemon juice mixture over carrots several times. Transfer to a serving platter. Sprinkle with pomegranate seeds. Season with black pepper.

Thanksgiving Tabbouleh Salad

INGREDIENTS

1/2 cup chopped shallots

1 clove garlic, minced

3 cups low-sodium vegetable broth

2 cups dry bulgur

1 12- to 16-oz. package chopped fresh butternut
squash

1 large cucumber, chopped (21/2 cups)

2 cups thinly sliced kale leaves, stems removed

1/2 cup dried tart cherries or cranberries

1/2 cup chopped fresh cilantro

1 teaspoon lime zest

1/2 cup lime juice

2 teaspoons pure maple syrup

2 teaspoons Dijon mustard

Sea salt, to taste

Freshly ground black pepper, to taste

INSTRUCTIONS

In a large saucepan cook shallots and garlic over medium 2 to 3 minutes, stirring occasionally and adding water, 1 to 2 tablespoons at a time, as needed to prevent sticking. Add vegetable broth, bulgur, and 2 cups water. Bring to boiling; reduce heat. Cover and simmer 15 to 20 minutes or until bulgur is tender. Drain any remaining liquid. Cool completely. (Bulgur can be transferred to an airtight container and refrigerated up to 3 days.)

Meanwhile, steam butternut squash according to package directions, about 7 minutes. Cool completely.

In a large bowl combine bulgur, squash, cucumber, kale, cherries, and cilantro. In a small bowl whisk together lime zest, lime juice, maple syrup, and Dijon mustard. Add half of the dressing to salad and toss to coat. Season with salt and pepper. Stir remaining dressing into salad just before serving.

Mexican-Style Brown Rice

INGREDIENTS

11/4 cups dry long grain brown rice, rinsed and drained

1 cup finely chopped yellow onion

8 cloves garlic, minced

1 teaspoon dried Mexican oregano, crushed

11/2 cups fresh or frozen green peas

1/2 cup finely chopped carrot

1 8-oz. can tomato sauce (3/4 cup)

2 tablespoons finely chopped fresh cilantro

Sea salt, to taste

INSTRUCTIONS

In a large saucepan combine rice, onion, garlic, and oregano. Cook over medium-low 10 minutes or until onion is softened and rice is toasted. (There should be enough moisture from the onion and rinsed rice to prevent burning.) Stir in peas, carrot, tomato sauce, and 2 cups water. Bring to boiling;

reduce heat. Cover and simmer 25 to 30 minutes or until rice is tender and water is absorbed. Turn off heat; let stand, covered, 10 minutes.

Uncover pan. Stir in cilantro and season with salt. Use a fork to fluff the rice and combine **Ingredients**.

Quinoa Tabbouleh with Pomegranate Seeds

INGREDIENTS

4 cups fresh parsley leaves (about 2 bunches)

2 cups cooked quinoa

1 cup cherry tomatoes, halved

1 Persian cucumber, cut into 1/2-inch dice (1 cup)

1 cup pomegranate arils

1 cup thinly sliced scallions

3 tablespoons lemon juice

Sea salt, to taste

Freshly ground black pepper, to taste

INSTRUCTIONS

In a food processor pulse parsley to the size of rice grains.

In a medium bowl stir together parsley and the remaining **Ingredients**. Taste and adjust seasoning. Serve at room temperature or chilled.

Lemony Spelt Salad with Roasted Broccolini

INGREDIENTS

3 lemons

1 lb. Broccolini

3 shallots, quartered

3 tablespoons pure maple syrup

1 tablespoon Dijon mustard

2 cloves garlic, minced

1 teaspoon grated fresh ginger

1/4 teaspoon sea salt

1/4 teaspoon freshly ground black pepper

5 cups cooled cooked spelt berries

2 15-oz. cans no-salt-added butter beans, rinsed
and drained (3 cups)

1/4 cup chopped fresh parsley

INSTRUCTIONS

Preheat oven to 425°F. Thinly slice 1 lemon. In a 15×10-inch baking pan arrange lemon slices, broccolini, and shallots in a single layer. Sprinkle with 2 tablespoons of water. Roast 15 to 20 minutes or until broccolini is crisp-tender and lightly browned.

Meanwhile, for dressing, remove 1 teaspoon zest and squeeze ⅓ cup juice from the remaining 2 lemons. Place in a large bowl with the next six **Ingredients** (through pepper) and 3 tablespoons water; whisk to combine. Reserve 2 tablespoons of dressing. Add spelt and beans to remaining dressing; toss to combine.

Drizzle roasted Broccolini, shallots, and lemon slices with the reserved dressing; toss to coat.

Arrange spelt mixture in a serving dish. Top with Broccolini mixture. Sprinkle with parsley.

Moroccan Carrot-Beet Salad

INGREDIENTS

1 orange

1 tablespoon lemon juice

1 tablespoon chopped fresh cilantro

1 tablespoon chopped fresh parsley

1/2 teaspoon flaxseed meal or chia seeds

1/4 teaspoon ground cumin

1/4 teaspoon ground coriander

1/8 teaspoon freshly ground black pepper

1 cup grated carrot

1 cup grated scrubbed beet

1 cup chopped seeded cucumber

1/2 cup finely chopped red onion

4 cups fresh baby spinach or salad greens

1 tablespoon golden raisins

1 tablespoon shelled roasted pistachios

Sea salt, to taste

INSTRUCTIONS

To make orange supremes, slice off ends of orange. Stand orange on a flat end. Slice off all the peel and bitter white pith in vertical strips, following the curve of the fruit. Working over a bowl to catch juice, slice between a membrane and section toward the center of the fruit. Repeat on the other side of the section, releasing it into the bowl.

In a medium bowl combine the next seven **Ingredients** (through pepper). Mix well. Add orange supremes and juice and the next four ingredients (through onion). Toss to combine.

Just before serving, arrange spinach on a platter. Top with carrot mixture, raisins, and pistachios. Season with salt.

Roasted Eggplant and Buckwheat Groats Fattoush

INGREDIENTS

2 whole wheat pita bread rounds, torn into 1- to 2-inch pieces

1 medium eggplant, cut into 2-inch cubes (6 cups)

2 red bell peppers, cut into thick strips

1 medium sweet onion, cut into thin wedges

6 tablespoons apple cider vinegar

1 cup oil-free hummus

1 teaspoon ground sumac

1 teaspoon Aleppo pepper

5 cups cooked buckwheat groats (kasha)

1 cup chopped cucumber

1/2 cup chopped fresh parsley

12 large romaine leaves

2 tablespoons chopped toasted walnuts

INSTRUCTIONS

Preheat oven to 400°F. On a baking sheet arrange pita pieces in a single layer. Bake 6 to 8 minutes or until toasted. Let cool.

In a 15×10-inch baking pan arrange eggplant, bell peppers, and onion. Drizzle with 2 tablespoons of the vinegar; toss to coat. Roast 30 to 35 minutes or until tender and lightly browned, stirring once. Transfer vegetables to a cutting board and coarsely chop.

Meanwhile, in a large bowl whisk together the remaining 1/4 cup vinegar, the hummus, sumac, and Aleppo pepper.

Add pita pieces, roasted vegetables, buckwheat groats, cucumber, and parsley to hummus mixture. Toss to combine. Spoon groats mixture into romaine leaves. Sprinkle with walnuts

Spiralized Daikon and Sweet Potato Noodles

INGREDIENTS

1 14-oz. package firm tofu

12 oz. daikon radishes, peeled

1 8-oz. sweet potato, peeled

2 tablespoons low-sodium tamari

1 tablespoon packed brown sugar

3 tablespoons lime juice

5 cloves garlic, minced

1 teaspoon grated fresh ginger

1 teaspoon Korean chili flakes (gochugaru)

3 tablespoons tahini

2 tablespoons chopped fresh cilantro

11/2 cups small broccoli florets

1 red bell pepper, cut into thin strips

1 cup matchstick-cut carrots

11/2 cups chopped fresh mango

1/4 cup thinly sliced scallions

Lime wedges

INSTRUCTIONS

Cut tofu block in half crosswise. Place tofu on a plate lined with a clean kitchen towel or a double layer of paper towels. Top with three more paper towels and a second plate. Weigh down top plate with something heavy, such as two 15-oz. cans of beans, and let stand 15 minutes to drain.

Preheat oven to 400°F. Line a baking sheet with parchment paper. Cut drained tofu into 1/2-inch cubes. Spread on prepared baking sheet. Bake 15 to 20 minutes or until golden.

Meanwhile, using the thick noodle blade on a vegetable spiral slicer, cut radishes and sweet potato into noodles. Cut noodles to desired length.

In a small bowl stir together tamari, brown sugar, 1 tablespoon lime juice, 4 cloves minced garlic, ginger, and Korean chili flakes. Set aside.

For Tahini-Lime Sauce, in a bowl stir together the tahini, the remaining 2 tablespoons lime juice, the remaining garlic, and the cilantro. Stir in water, 1 tablespoon at a time, as needed to reach drizzling consistency.

In an extra-large nonstick skillet cover and cook radish and sweet potato noodles, broccoli, bell pepper, and carrots over medium-high 8 to 10 minutes or until crisp-tender, stirring frequently and adding water, 1 to 2 tablespoons at a time, as needed to prevent sticking. Add tofu and the tamari mixture. Cook 2 to 3 minutes or until heated through, tossing gently. Spoon mixture into bowls. Top with mango and drizzle with Tahini-Lime Sauce. Sprinkle with scallions and serve with lime wedges.

HALLELUJAH DIET RECIPES FOR SOUP AND STEW

Pinto Bean and Hominy Soup

INGREDIENTS

1 cup chopped onion

6 cloves garlic, minced

4 cups low-sodium vegetable broth

2 15-oz. cans no-salt-added pinto beans, rinsed and drained (3 cups)

2 15-oz. cans golden and/or white hominy, rinsed and drained (3 cups)

1 cup chopped orange bell pepper

1 tablespoon mild or hot chili powder

2 teaspoon dried oregano, crushed

1 teaspoon ground cumin

1/4 teaspoon freshly ground black pepper

⅓ cup chopped fresh cilantro, plus more for garnish

1/2 cup Tofu Sour Cream

1 avocado, halved, seeded, peeled, and chopped

1/4 cup finely chopped red onion

Lime wedges

INSTRUCTIONS

Set a 6-quart electric multicooker to sauté setting. Add onion and garlic. Cook 5 minutes, stirring occasionally and adding broth, 1 tablespoon at a time, as needed to prevent sticking. Add remaining broth and the next seven **Ingredients** (through black pepper).

Lock lid in place; set pressure valve to sealing. Set cooker on high pressure to cook 2 minutes. Let stand to release pressure naturally (about 15 minutes). Carefully release any remaining pressure. Open lid carefully. Stir in cilantro.

Top servings with Tofu Sour Cream, avocado, and red onion. Garnish with additional cilantro and serve with lime wedges.

Creamy Vegetable Soup with Escarole

INGREDIENTS

11/2 cups chopped carrots

11/2 cups sliced fresh mushrooms

1 cup chopped celery

1 cup chopped onion

1 cup frozen corn

1 tablespoon minced garlic

4 cups low-sodium vegetable broth

11/4 teaspoon dried thyme, crushed

11/4 teaspoon dried dill, crushed

6 oz. dry whole wheat rotini pasta

4 cups coarsely chopped fresh escarole or endive

1 15-oz. can no-salt-added chickpeas, undrained

2 teaspoons lemon zest

3 tablespoons lemon juice

Sea salt, to taste

Freshly ground black pepper, to taste

Crusty whole grain French bread (optional)

INSTRUCTIONS

In a large pot cook the first six ingredients (through garlic) over medium 6 minutes, stirring occasionally and adding broth, 1 to 2 tablespoons at a time, as needed to prevent sticking. Add the remaining broth, the thyme, and dill. Bring to boiling. Stir in rotini and escarole. Return to boiling; reduce heat. Cook, uncovered, 8 to 10 minutes or until rotini is tender.

Place chickpeas in a small blender or food processor. Cover and blend until very smooth, adding a small amount of water if needed. Add to soup with lemon zest and juice; mix well.

Season with salt and pepper. Serve with crusty bread (if using).

Curried Sweet Potato Soup

INGREDIENTS

21/2 lb. sweet potatoes, peeled and cut into 2-inch wedges or chunks

2 large red bell peppers, cut into big chunks

1 medium yellow onion, cut into 2-inch wedges or pieces

6 cloves garlic

4 cups low-sodium vegetable broth

1/2 teaspoon curry powder

1/4 to 1/2 teaspoon crushed red pepper

11/2 teaspoon apple cider vinegar

Sea salt, to taste

1 tablespoon pumpkin seeds

INSTRUCTIONS

Preheat oven to 375°F. Line two baking sheets with parchment paper. Spread sweet potatoes, bell peppers, onion, and garlic on prepared baking sheets. Bake 40 minutes or until potatoes are tender.

Transfer baked vegetables to a blender; add broth. Cover and blend until smooth. (Blend in batches, if necessary.) Transfer to a large pot. Stir in curry powder and crushed red pepper. Bring to boiling; reduce heat. Simmer, uncovered, 10 minutes to blend flavors.

Stir in vinegar and season with salt. Top servings with pumpkin seeds and additional crushed red pepper.

Veggie Jambalaya with Black-Eyed Peas

INGREDIENTS

1⅓ cups dry brown rice

1 cup chopped onion

1 cup chopped green bell pepper

1 cup chopped celery

1/2 cup no-salt-added tomato paste

2 tablespoons salt-free Cajun seasoning

2 15-oz. cans no-salt-added black- eyed peas, rinsed and drained

2 14.5-oz. cans no-salt-added diced tomatoes, undrained

2 cups low-sodium vegetable broth

1/2 teaspoon smoked paprika

Sea salt, to taste

Freshly ground black pepper, to taste

1/4 cup sliced scallions

1/4 cup chopped fresh parsley

Hot pepper sauce (optional)

INSTRUCTIONS

In a large saucepan combine rice and 4 cups water. Bring to boiling; reduce heat. Cover and simmer 30 minutes or until rice is nearly tender.

Meanwhile, in a large pot cook onion, bell pepper, and celery over medium 5 minutes, stirring occasionally and adding water, 1 to 2 tablespoons at a time, as needed to prevent sticking. Add tomato paste and Cajun seasoning; cook and stir 1 minute. Add black-eyed peas, tomatoes, broth, and paprika. Bring to boiling; reduce heat. Simmer, uncovered, 30 minutes. Drain any water from the rice; add rice to vegetables. Cook 15 minutes more or until jambalaya is thick. Season with salt and black pepper. Sprinkle with scallions and parsley. If desired, serve with hot sauce.

Roasted Kabocha Squash and Veggie Stew

INGREDIENTS

4 cups cubed peeled kabocha squash (3/4-inch cubes)

4 medium carrots, halved lengthwise and thickly sliced (2 cups)

8 oz. fresh cremini mushrooms, halved

1 medium fennel bulb, quartered, cored, and cut into 1/4-inch wedges

1/4 cup white wine vinegar

1 cup chopped onion

4 cloves garlic, minced

4 cups low-sodium vegetable broth

2 tablespoons no-salt-added tomato paste

1 teaspoon dried Italian seasoning, crushed

4 cups shredded fresh Swiss chard

Sea salt, to taste

Freshly ground black pepper, to taste

2 cups hot cooked farro

1/2 cup slivered fresh basil

2 tablespoons toasted pine nuts, chopped

INSTRUCTIONS

Preheat oven to 400°F. Line two large shallow baking pans with parchment paper or foil. Arrange squash and carrots in one baking pan and mushrooms and fennel in the other baking pan. Sprinkle all vegetables with vinegar. Roast 30 minutes or until just tender and lightly browned, stirring once.

In a 4- to 6-quart pot cook onion in 2 tablespoons water over medium 4 minutes or until tender, stirring occasionally and adding water, 1 to 2 tablespoons at a time, as needed to prevent sticking. Add garlic; cook 1 minute. Add roasted vegetables, broth, tomato paste, and Italian seasoning. Bring to boiling; reduce heat. Cover and simmer 15 minutes, stirring occasionally. Stir in chard until wilted. Season with salt and pepper.

Stir together farro, basil, and pine nuts. Spoon into bowls. Top with stew.

Vegan Taco Soup

INGREDIENTS

8 cups quartered roma tomatoes

1 cup coarsely chopped onion

2 poblano chiles, halved and seeded

1 jalapeño chile, halved and seeded

6 cloves garlic

2 teaspoons dried oregano, crushed

1 teaspoon pure cane sugar

1/4 teaspoon crushed red pepper (optional)

3 cups low-sodium vegetable broth

2 cups frozen roasted corn

1 15-oz. can no-salt-added black beans, undrained

1 14- to 20-oz. can no-salt-added jackfruit, drained and shredded

Sea salt, to taste

2 6-inch corn tortillas, cut into strips

1/2 cup chopped fresh cilantro

Lime wedges

INSTRUCTIONS

Preheat oven to 450°F. Line two 15×10-inch baking pans with foil. In a large bowl combine the first eight ingredients (through crushed red pepper, if using); mix well. Spread evenly in pans. Roast 45 minutes or until charred in places; cool slightly. Transfer to a blender. (You may want to work in batches.) Cover and blend until nearly smooth. Transfer soup base to a large saucepan. Reduce oven temperature to 400°F.

Stir broth, corn, undrained beans, and jackfruit into soup base. Bring mixture to boiling; reduce heat. Simmer, uncovered, 10 minutes to blend flavors, stirring occasionally. Season with salt.

Meanwhile, spread tortilla strips on a baking sheet. Bake 5 minutes or until crisp.

Serve soup topped with cilantro, tortilla strips, and, if you like, sliced additional jalapeño. Serve lime wedges on the side.

Green Cabbage and White Bean Soup

INGREDIENTS

2 lb. green cabbage, cored and cut into 1-inch pieces (4 cups)

1 cup finely chopped leek, white part only

1 cup chopped carrots

6 cloves garlic, minced

1 bay leaf

11/2 teaspoons dried Italian seasoning, crushed

1 15-oz. can white beans (any variety), rinsed and drained

1/4 cup tomato paste

1 tablespoon brown rice vinegar

1/4 teaspoon freshly ground black pepper

Sea salt, to taste

1 tablespoon finely chopped fresh parsley

INSTRUCTIONS

In a large pot combine the first six ingredients (through Italian seasoning) and 1/4 cup water. Cook over medium about 10 minutes or until carrots are tender, stirring frequently and adding water, 1 to 2 tablespoons at a time, as needed to prevent sticking.

Add beans, tomato paste, and 6 cups water to pot. Bring to boiling; reduce heat. Simmer, uncovered, 5 to 7 minutes more or until thickened. Remove and discard bay leaf. Stir in vinegar, pepper, and salt. Sprinkle with parsley.

Vegan Pasta Fagioli

INGREDIENTS

4 roma tomatoes, cut into large pieces

2 cups dry whole wheat pasta, such as penne, fusilli, or shells

1 tablespoon garlic powder

1 tablespoon onion powder

1 tablespoon dried Italian seasoning, crushed

2 cups frozen vegetable medley of your choice

1 15-oz. can chickpeas, rinsed and drained (11/2 cups)

1/8 teaspoon freshly ground black pepper

1 tablespoon white wine vinegar

Sea salt, to taste

INSTRUCTIONS

In a blender combine tomatoes and 1 cup water. Cover and blend to desired texture. Transfer to a large pot and add 5 cups water. Bring to boiling. Stir in pasta, garlic powder, onion powder, and Italian seasoning. Reduce heat to medium; simmer 5 minutes. (Pasta will be about halfway cooked.)

Stir in frozen vegetables and chickpeas. Return to boiling; reduce heat. Simmer 8 to 10 minutes more or until pasta is tender. Stir in pepper and vinegar;

season with salt. Cook 2 minutes more to allow flavors to blend. Serve warm.

Creamy Carrot and Pea Soup

INGREDIENTS

2 cups chopped onion

3 cloves garlic, minced

3 cups chopped carrots

1 tablespoon grated fresh ginger

1 32-oz. package low-sodium vegetable broth

3 cups chopped peeled Yukon gold potatoes

1 teaspoon ground coriander

Dash ground cinnamon

2 15-oz. cans no-salt-added chickpeas, rinsed and drained (3 cups)

2 cups unsweetened coconut milk beverage (do not use canned)

2 tablespoons lime juice

Sea salt, to taste

Freshly ground black pepper, to taste

2 cups fresh sugar snap peas, halved

INSTRUCTIONS

In a large pot cook onion and garlic over medium 5 minutes, stirring occasionally and adding water, 1 to 2 tablespoons at a time, as needed to prevent sticking. Add carrots and ginger; cook 3 to 4 minutes, adding water, 1 to 2 tablespoons at a time, as needed to prevent sticking. Do not let the ginger burn.

Add vegetable broth, potatoes, coriander, and cinnamon. Bring to boiling; reduce heat. Cover and simmer 15 to 20 minutes or until potatoes are very tender.

Add chickpeas. Remove from heat. Using an immersion blender, puree soup until very smooth. (Or transfer in batches to a blender; cover and blend until smooth. Return to pot.) Stir in coconut milk; simmer 5 minutes. Add lime juice. Season with salt and pepper.

Place sugar snap peas in a steamer basket in a large saucepan. Add water to saucepan to just below basket. Bring to boiling. Steam, covered, 1 to 2 minutes or just until tender. Add to soup, reserving a few to garnish servings.

Lemon Orzo Soup with Jackfruit

INGREDIENTS

2 cups chopped onion

1 cup chopped celery

3 cloves garlic, minced

2 teaspoons grated fresh ginger

1 32-oz. package low-sodium vegetable broth

2 cups sliced carrots

1 14.5-oz. can green jackfruit, rinsed, drained, and shredded

2 teaspoons lemon zest

6 oz. dry whole wheat orzo

1 15-oz. can no-salt-added navy beans, rinsed and drained (11/2 cups)

1/4 cup chopped fresh parsley

2 tablespoons lemon juice

Sea salt, to taste

Freshly ground black pepper, to taste

INSTRUCTIONS

In a large pot cook onion, celery, garlic, and ginger over medium 4 minutes, stirring occasionally and adding water, 1 to 2 tablespoons at a time, as needed to prevent sticking. Add vegetable broth, carrots, jackfruit, lemon zest, and 2 cups water. Bring to boiling; reduce heat. Cover and simmer 5 minutes.

Stir in orzo; cook 8 to 10 minutes or until orzo is tender. Stir in beans and parsley. Add lemon juice. Season with salt and pepper.

Toni Okamoto's Sopa de Fideo

INGREDIENTS

1/2 medium yellow onion, diced

3 medium garlic cloves, minced

1 small zucchini, diced

1 (7-ounce) package whole wheat angel hair pasta, broken into small pieces

2 Roma tomatoes, diced

11/2 teaspoons ground cumin

5 cups vegetable broth

1 (8-ounce) can tomato sauce

INSTRUCTIONS

In a medium saucepan, heat 1/4 cup water over medium-high heat. Sauté the onion and garlic in it for 1 minute. Add the zucchini and pasta and sauté until the noodles turn very light brown, 1 to 2 minutes.

Add the tomatoes, cumin, broth, and tomato sauce and stir until thoroughly combined.

Bring to a boil, cover with a lid, reduce the heat to low, and let simmer until the pasta has softened, about 10 minutes.

Lentil and Spinach Soup

INGREDIENTS

1 cup dry brown or green lentils, rinsed and drained

1/2 cup finely chopped onion

6 cloves garlic, minced

6 cups low-sodium vegetable broth

2 teaspoons chopped fresh thyme

2 teaspoons chopped fresh oregano

2 cups chopped peeled butternut squash

1 cup finely chopped tomato

1/4 teaspoon crushed red pepper

2 tablespoons lemon juice

Sea salt, to taste

Freshly ground black pepper, to taste

6 cups packed fresh spinach, chopped

1 tablespoon lemon zest

INSTRUCTIONS

In a bowl combine lentils and 3 cups hot water. Let soak at least 20 minutes.

Heat a large saucepan over medium. Add onion, garlic, and 1/4 cup water. Cook 10 minutes or until onion is tender, stirring occasionally.

Drain lentils; add to saucepan along with vegetable broth, thyme, and oregano. Bring to boiling; reduce heat. Cover and simmer 20 minutes. Stir in squash, tomato, and crushed red pepper. Cover and cook 20 minutes more or until squash is tender. Stir in lemon juice. Season with salt and black pepper.

Stir in spinach and lemon zest. Cook 1 to 2 minutes more or until spinach wilts slightly. Serve immediately.

Shiro Wat (Chickpea Flour Stew)

INGREDIENTS

1 cup chickpea flour

1 cup chopped red onion

12 cloves garlic, minced

1 cup chopped tomato

11/2 tablespoons Berbere Spice Blend

1/2 teaspoon ground cardamom

1 teaspoon tahini or cashew butter

2 tablespoons lemon juice

Sea salt, to taste

INSTRUCTIONS

Heat a large nonstick skillet over medium-low. Add chickpea flour; cook for 10-15 minutes or until flour releases a toasted aroma, stirring frequently. Transfer to a large bowl; let cool.

In a large saucepan combine onion, garlic, and 1/4 cup water. Cover and cook over medium 10 minutes or until onion is tender, stirring occasionally. Add tomato, Berbere Spice Blend, and cardamom; cook 10 minutes more.

Add tahini, lemon juice, and 6 cups water to the toasted chickpea flour; whisk until smooth. Add mixture to pan with onion mixture. Bring mixture to boiling; reduce heat. Cover and cook 30 minutes or until stew is thickened, stirring occasionally. Season with salt.

Winter Squash Soup with Pistachio Gremolata

INGREDIENTS

1 cup chopped onion

6 cloves garlic, minced

5 cups low-sodium vegetable broth

3 cups 1-inch cubed peeled butternut squash

1 1-lb. delicata squash, halved, seeded, and cut into 1-inch pieces (3 cups)

1 fennel bulb, cored and chopped (2 cups)

1 15-oz. can no-salt-added tomato sauce

1 14.5-oz. can fire-roasted diced tomatoes

1 cup chopped red bell pepper

2 teaspoons Italian seasoning, crushed

1/2 teaspoon crushed red pepper

12 oz. dry whole wheat cavatappi, rotini, or bow-tie pasta

1 15-oz. can no-salt-added cannellini beans, rinsed and drained (11/2 cups)

1/4 teaspoon sea salt

1/2 cup chopped fresh flat-leaf parsley

⅓ cup chopped pistachio nuts

1 teaspoon lemon zest

INSTRUCTIONS

Set a 6-quart electric multicooker to sauté setting. Add onion and garlic. Cook 5 minutes, stirring occasionally and adding broth, 1 tablespoon at a time, as needed to prevent sticking. Add remaining broth and the next eight **Ingredients** (through crushed red pepper).

Lock lid in place; set pressure valve to sealing. Set cooker on high pressure to cook 8 minutes. Carefully quick-release pressure according to manufacturer's directions. Open lid carefully.

Meanwhile, cook pasta according to package directions. Stir cooked pasta, the beans, and salt into soup. Cover and let stand 5 minutes. For gremolata, stir together parsley, pistachios, and lemon zest. Top servings with gremolata.

Caribbean Sweet Potato Stew

INGREDIENTS

11/2 cup chopped onion

1 cup coarsely chopped carrots

1 fresh poblano chile, seeded and chopped (1 cup)

3/4 cup chopped red bell pepper

1 cup chopped celery

2 teaspoons curry powder

2 teaspoons grated fresh ginger

1/2 teaspoon ground allspice

2 lb. sweet potatoes, peeled if desired, cut into 1-inch cubes (6 cups)

4 cups low-sodium vegetable broth

1 15-oz. can no-salt-added black beans, rinsed and drained (11/2 cups)

1 14.5-oz. can no-salt-added diced tomatoes

Sea salt, to taste

Freshly ground black pepper, to taste

2 cups packed fresh cilantro

1 cup packed fresh parsley

1/2 cup chopped celery

1/2 cup chopped scallions

8 cloves garlic

1 fresh fresno chile, seeded and very finely chopped

2 cups hot cooked brown rice

2 tablespoons toasted coconut (optional)

Lime wedges

INSTRUCTIONS

In a Dutch oven cook 1 cup onion, the carrots, poblano chile, bell pepper, and 1/2 cup celery over medium for 5 minutes or until carrots are softened and other vegetables are tender, stirring occasionally and adding water, 1 to 2 tablespoons at a time, as needed to prevent sticking. Add curry powder, 1 teaspoon ginger, and allspice; cook and stir 1 minute. Stir in sweet potatoes, broth, beans, and undrained tomatoes. Bring to boiling; reduce heat. Cover and simmer 20 to 25 minutes or until sweet potatoes are tender. Season with salt and black pepper.

For Caribbean Green Sauce, in a blender or food processor combine cilantro, parsley, the remaining 1/2 cup onion and 1/2 cup celery, scallions, garlic, and remaining 1 teaspoon ginger. Cover and blend, adding water 1 tablespoon at a time until almost smooth. Stir in fresno chile (if desired). Sauce can be transferred to an airtight container and stored in the refrigerator up to 5 days.

Stir ⅓ cup of the Caribbean Green Sauce into hot cooked rice. Serve stew in bowls over rice. If desired, top with additional green sauce and sprinkle with toasted coconut. Serve with lime wedges.

CHAPTER 6: WHY THE HALLELUJAH DIET IS PERFECT FOR YOU

The Hallelujah Diet adopts a comprehensive approach to health and well-being by advocating for a raw food, plant-based dietary regimen. Rooted in biblical principles, this diet underscores the notion that a balanced diet not only fosters physical vitality but also nurtures spiritual well-being by providing the body with vital nutrients sourced from a diverse array of fruits, vegetables, nuts, and seeds. Central to this dietary philosophy is the Hallelujah Plate, a visual guide that encourages a nourishing blend of fresh, leafy greens, fruits, and nuts and seeds, promoting a harmonious relationship between food consumption and overall health.

In addition to emphasizing nutritional balance, the Hallelujah Diet incorporates unique strategies to support the body's innate detoxification processes. These include cleansing rituals, periodic juice fasts, and intermittent fasting, all aimed at enhancing the body's natural ability to eliminate toxins and promote optimal health. In instances where specific nutritional deficiencies may arise, supplements are recommended, with a focus on essential elements such as vitamin B12, iron, calcium, and omega-3 fatty acids to address potential gaps in dietary intake.

Beyond dietary considerations, the Hallelujah Diet underscores the importance of holistic wellness practices encompassing physical, mental, and spiritual dimensions. This includes prioritizing regular exercise, cultivating relaxation through practices like meditation and prayer, ensuring adequate sleep, and fostering positive social connections. Spiritual wellness is further emphasized through practices such as prayer, reflection, and gratitude, all aimed at deepening the connection between food choices and spiritual development.

While the Hallelujah Diet offers a holistic perspective on health, it acknowledges the individuality of each person's tastes and dietary needs. Achieving a healthy equilibrium requires careful consideration of one's health goals, responsible supplementation, and mindful fasting practices. Consulting with a healthcare professional before making significant changes to one's diet or lifestyle is strongly recommended to ensure that the Hallelujah Diet aligns with individual health needs and objectives. By collaborating with a healthcare provider, individuals can embark on a journey towards achieving physical, mental, and spiritual wellness through the principles of the Hallelujah Diet.

Detoxification and Fasting in the Hallelujah Diet

As an integral part of its comprehensive approach to health and wellness, the Hallelujah Diet incorporates fasting and cleansing as fundamental elements. Fasting holds both spiritual and culinary significance, rooted in the belief that abstaining from certain foods for designated periods can facilitate cleansing and detoxification processes within the body. Intermittent fasting, as well as occasional extended fasts, are common practices embraced by adherents of the Hallelujah Diet.

Intermittent fasting can be likened to a revolving door between periods of eating and abstaining from food. Proponents of this method suggest that it induces cellular regeneration and purification by prompting the body into a state of rest and repair during fasting intervals. Some individuals opt for prolonged fasting periods, lasting 24 or 48 hours, while others adhere to daily time-restricted eating windows.

In tandem with fasting, the Hallelujah Diet incorporates cleansing rituals to support the body's innate detoxification mechanisms. This may entail increasing fluid intake and consuming specific cleansing foods, such as detoxifying fruits and vegetables. The prevailing belief is that these practices aid in enhancing overall health by facilitating the elimination of accumulated toxins from the body.

Juice fasting is particularly promoted by the Hallelujah Diet as an effective means of cleansing the body. Many proponents attest to the superior absorption of nutrients from freshly squeezed vegetable juices. Juice fasts typically involve consuming only fresh juices for a designated period, providing the digestive system with a respite while supplying essential nutrients to the body.

It is important to exercise caution and consider individual health needs when engaging in cleansing practices such as fasting. Prior to embarking on any fasting or cleansing regimen, it is advisable for individuals who are pregnant, nursing, have underlying medical conditions, or are taking medications to consult with their healthcare providers. Responsible and informed participation is paramount to reaping the health benefits associated with the Hallelujah Diet's fasting and cleansing protocols.

Practices of Daily Living and Spiritual Well-Being

Embracing a holistic approach to overall well-being that encompasses spiritual wellness, the lifestyle practices advocated by the Hallelujah Diet extend beyond mere dietary considerations. The regimen recognizes the interconnectedness of physical, emotional, and spiritual health, emphasizing various lifestyle activities to promote a comprehensive sense of wellness.

Regular physical exercise is widely acknowledged as a cornerstone of a healthy lifestyle. Many individuals attest to the transformative effects of consistent physical activity on their health and vitality. According to prevailing wisdom, regular exercise enhances various physiological processes, facilitates improved blood circulation, and contributes to psychological and emotional well-being. Aligned with the Hallelujah Diet's commitment to holistic living, it encourages participation in exercises that enhance flexibility, strength, and cardiovascular health, thereby fostering a well-rounded approach to physical fitness.

Stress management is another pivotal aspect of the lifestyle advocated by the Hallelujah Diet. Recognizing the profound impact of stress on both physical and spiritual health, the regimen emphasizes the importance of cultivating inner calm and resilience. Practices such as mindfulness, meditation, and prayer are recommended as effective means of alleviating stress and promoting spiritual peace. By reducing stress levels, individuals are believed to enhance the body's inherent healing mechanisms, thereby facilitating overall well-being.

Adequate sleep is also prioritized within the framework of the Hallelujah Diet's lifestyle recommendations. Acknowledging the critical role of sleep in facilitating physical and mental rejuvenation, the regimen underscores the importance of establishing regular sleep patterns and ensuring sufficient rest. By prioritizing restorative sleep, individuals are believed to enhance energy levels and support overall health and vitality.

Furthermore, the Hallelujah Diet underscores the significance of nurturing supportive relationships and fostering community engagement. Spiritual well-being is perceived as intimately linked to interpersonal connections and a sense of belonging within a supportive community. By cultivating meaningful relationships and actively participating in community life, individuals are believed to enhance their spiritual health and experience a sense of connectedness and support on their wellness journey.

Rooted in religious principles, the Hallelujah Diet emphasizes the integration of spiritual practices into daily life. Practices such as prayer, contemplation, and gratitude are recommended as means of fostering spiritual growth and alignment with divine principles. Founder Reverend George Malkmus underscores the importance of aligning dietary choices with biblical teachings, recognizing the integral connection between physical and spiritual health.

In summary, the Hallelujah Diet transcends conventional dietary paradigms to encompass a holistic way of life that encompasses exercise, relaxation, social connection, spiritual well-being, and stress management. At its core, this comprehensive approach is grounded in the belief that a harmonious lifestyle fosters total well-being, striving to empower individuals to achieve optimal physical and spiritual health.

CHAPTER 7: FINAL THOUGHTS

In wrapping up our exploration of the Hallelujah Diet, it becomes abundantly clear that this lifestyle transcends mere dietary guidelines, encapsulating a holistic philosophy that encompasses the entirety of human existence. Throughout the pages of this book, we've delved into the multifaceted layers of the Hallelujah Diet, uncovering its dietary precepts, lifestyle recommendations, and spiritual ethos.

At its essence, the Hallelujah Diet represents a profound paradigm shift—a departure from conventional dietary practices towards a more comprehensive approach to well-being. Beyond the realm of nutrition, it beckons individuals to embark on a journey towards holistic health, addressing not only the physical aspects of wellness but also the emotional, mental, and spiritual dimensions of human existence.

Central to the Hallelujah Diet is the recognition of the interconnectedness of body, mind, and spirit—a fundamental principle that underpins its dietary guidelines and lifestyle prescriptions. Through the integration of physical activity, stress management techniques, restorative sleep, nurturing relationships, and spiritual practices, the Hallelujah Diet offers a blueprint for achieving optimal health and vitality in every facet of life.

Rooted in deeply held religious beliefs, the Hallelujah Diet invites individuals to align their dietary choices with spiritual principles, fostering a deeper connection with their faith and a greater sense of purpose and meaning. Founder Reverend George Malkmus's unwavering commitment to the spiritual dimension of health underscores the profound impact that faith and spirituality can have on one's overall well-being.

As we conclude our exploration of the Hallelujah Diet, let us reflect on the transformative power of this holistic lifestyle approach. May it serve as a beacon of hope and inspiration, guiding us towards a life of abundance, vitality, and wholeness. By embracing the principles of the Hallelujah Diet, may we embark on a journey of self-discovery and self-realization, finding fulfillment and joy in every aspect of our lives.

In the journey ahead, may the principles of the Hallelujah Diet serve as a guiding light, illuminating the path towards total well-being and empowering us to live our lives to the fullest.